ALSO BY DANIEL G. AMEN, M.D.

Sex on the Brain

Change Your Brain, Change Your Life

Healing ADD

Preventing Alzheimer's (with William Rodman Shankle)

Healing Anxiety and Depression (with Lisa Routh)

Healing the Hardware of the Soul

Coaching Yourself to Success

New Skills for Frazzled Parents

What I Learned from a Penguin (with Jesse Payne)

The Amen Clinic Program
for Achieving and Sustaining
Optimal Mental Performance

THREE RIVERS PRESS • NEW YORK

MAKING A GOOD BRAIN GREAT

DANIEL G. AMEN, M.D.

Originally published in hardcover in the United States by Harmony Books, an imprint of the Crown
Publishing Group, a division of Random House, Inc., New York, in 2005.

Library of Congress Cataloging-in-Publication Data
Amen, Daniel G.
Making a good brain great : the Amen clinic program for achieving and sustaining
optimal mental performance / Daniel G. Amen.— 1st ed.
Includes bibliographical references.
1. Brain—Popular works.   2. Mental health—Popular works.   I. Title.
QP376.A4264 2005
612.8′2—dc22   2005006711

ISBN-13: 978-1-4000-8209-4
ISBN-10: 1-4000-8209-9

Printed in the United States of America

Design by Helene Berinsky

20 19 18 17 16 15 14 13 12

First Paperback Edition

CONTENTS

PART II

THE AMEN CLINIC PROGRAM FOR
MAKING A GOOD BRAIN GREAT

MAKING A GOOD BRAIN GREAT

MAKING A GOOD BRAIN GREAT

Learning how to make a good brain great, or a difficult one better, has been my passion for the last twenty years. Having scanned and worked with more than thirty thousand brains, more than any other living soul, it is very clear to me that the brain is involved in everything we do and everything we are. I have learned that when your brain works right, you work right, and that when your brain is troubled, you have trouble in your life. Brain health is essential to all aspects of the quality of life.

Your brain can be even better than it is right now—and I will show you how, step by step! Whether you are already functioning at a high level (at work, in your relationships, or within yourself) and want to keep it that way, or you are struggling to get through the day and need help, improving the inner workings of your brain is the most important first step to having the life you want.

I live in Newport Beach, California, which is a wonderful place, but it has the reputation for being home to the greatest number of plastic surgeons and for being what some would call a plastic society. What many people do not realize, when they go to a plastic surgeon to have their noses redone, their breasts enlarged, or their wrinkles alleviated, is that they still will be the same on the inside after the procedure is finished and the stitches removed. Change is much more effective from the inside out. My goal in this book is to teach you to love and care for your brain as much as you love and care for your skin, your belly, and your bottom. It sounds silly at first, but when you ponder it for a while, it makes perfect sense. To be your best self, you must have a brain that works at its best. This is what we strive to do at the Amen Clinics (in Newport Beach and Fairfield, California; Tacoma, Washington; and Reston, Virginia); we work hard to help balance the function of people's brains and improve their lives. Whether you are struggling in school, at work, at home, in relationships, or within yourself, the Amen Clinics work hard to help you to get the best brain and life function possible. Your brain and your life are inseparably linked.

The great news is that the brain is malleable and able to change. With targeted strategies, you can make a good brain great. But if you don't actively work out a plan to help it, the brain becomes significantly less active with age. Lower brain activity and blood flow causes people to have trouble remembering facts and names, they become more easily fatigued, they struggle to learn new information, and they are at greater risk for more serious problems, such as strokes or Alzheimer's disease as they move into their fifties, sixties, and seventies. Isn't it strange that most people are focused on taking care of their skin, weight, job, home, and pet, while ignoring the part of them that matters most? It doesn't have to be this way. This book is your guide to loving, caring, and nurturing your brain.

To show you what I mean, here are a few examples of the kinds of people who can benefit from the information in *Making a Good Brain Great*.

Bart, at forty-seven, is a very good doctor who has built a thriving practice. His patients and employees love him, and he is respected in the medical community. He has been working hard for many years, but he has not taken very good care of himself. He feels tired at the end of the day and doesn't have much energy for his wife and young children. In the last ten years, Bart has put on an extra fifteen pounds and doesn't feel quite as sharp as he once did. No one would notice his problems, but he can feel that he is clearly not his best self.

Angela, thirty-eight, owns a boutique dress shop. She is happy, energetic, and a good businesswoman. Her employees adore her, and she has been in a stable marriage for fifteen years. One of her concerns is that both her father and her mother suffered from memory problems in their sixties, and she fears those same problems will happen to her.

Marian, twenty-six, works at an ad agency. She is alternately "a star" and then "the problem" employee. At times she does wonderful work, and at other times she drives everyone crazy with her temper, moodiness, and unpredictability. She has been on the verge of being fired several times, but each time she pulled herself together and again did great work, for a while.

John, sixty-two, is a business professor at a major southern California university. Over the years he has been seen by others as successful, happy, and funny. After a seemingly minor fall from a ladder at his home two years ago, he just hasn't been himself. It has been hard for him to describe the difference, and no one else seems to notice it. For the first time he finds himself late grading papers, more distracted at meetings, and a bit more irritable with his wife.

What do Bart, Angela, Marian, and John have in common with one another and with millions of others? They are successful, competent people who need to optimize their own brain function to be at their best. Bart has an overworked, stressed, malnourished, and tired brain; Angela has a brain at risk for early dementia; Marian has a brain that has erratic storms of activity; and John hurt his brain in a fall. All their brains are functional, but they need to be tuned, balanced, and properly nourished to remain in excellent health. Without this regimen they are all at risk for brain deterioration that, although subtle, will rob them of their best abilities and potential.

Here are the basic principles that Bart, Angela, Marian, and John and the rest of us need to keep in mind.

- The brain is involved in everything you do. How you think, how you feel, how you act, and how well you get along with other people has to do with the moment-by-moment functioning of your brain.
- When your brain works right, you tend to be effective, thoughtful, creative, and energetic.
- When the brain is troubled, you may have problems with depression, anxiety, work performance, impulsivity, anger, inflexibility, memory, and relationships.
- Your brain dysfunction, even when subtle, may be getting in your way of success.
- Your brain has only so much reserve. A lifetime of abuse or neglect (smoking, too much caffeine or alcohol, drug abuse, brain injuries, excessive stress) all add up and take years of healthy mental functioning away from you.
- With the right plan, you can reverse damage and optimize your own brain and subsequently improve your life.

• You (and your brain) can be better than you are, even if you are already in good shape!

Making a Good Brain Great is a practical guide to understanding and optimizing the functioning in your own brain, so you can be the best person possible. It will also teach you how to enhance the brains of your children and those you love. Unfortunately, many of the things that we do as parents, partners, and friends that we think are loving, such as encouraging people to eat second helpings, are actually harmful to brain function.

The book is divided into two parts. Part I, a basic primer on the brain, will explain why it is essential to love and nurture the brain and how it is intimately involved in all you do. It outlines the nine basic principles of the Amen Clinics (Chapters 1–9). Part II contains the Amen Clinic Program for Making a Good Brain Great. These practical strategies and exercises are based on real-life experience with thousands of people. It will also teach you when and how to seek professional help if brain problems need more extensive evaluation and treatment, such as John's minor brain injury and Marian's emotional brain storms. The ultimate lesson in this book is for you to learn how to love, respect, and care for your brain, as you would love, respect, and care for a cherished child or grandchild. When you develop this deep sense of caring for your brain, you will be more likely to protect and nurture it, so that over time it will help you be effective in love, work, and all you do.

THE PROBLEM

Most people do not consider caring for their brain to be an essential aspect of good health. Even though you probably already accept the basic brain principles outlined above, individuals rarely think about the day-to-day health of their own brain. Until they came to our clinic, Bart, Angela, Marian, and John never gave their own brains much thought, or considered how they work or how to keep them healthy. It is rarer still for people to actively exercise and nourish them. Schools teach no required classes on practical brain science for everyday living, yet the brain is more important than geography, economics, algebra, literature, and world history combined. In fact, the brain is the place where all this knowledge lives.

Without much forethought, people pollute their brains with caffeine, cigarettes, alcohol, and drugs and by living in toxic cities. Without knowing they're doing it, they hurt their brains by hitting soccer balls with their heads, playing tackle football, snowboarding and skiing without helmets, or riding motorcycles (even with helmets). People stress their brains by working at an ever-frenzied pace, holding on to resentments from the past, not getting enough sleep, and driving in nightmare traffic. And without realizing it, people deprive the brain of proper nutrients, eating fast-food diets and not using appropriate supplements.

Brain dysfunction is the number-one reason people fail at school, at work, and in relationships. After all, the brain is the organ of learning, working, and loving. When the brain is ineffective, so are we.

THE PROMISE

By taking simple steps to balance and optimize your brain function, you will be able to enhance and take better control of your life. With appropriate forethought (using your brain), you can learn how to keep your brain healthy throughout life. My goal has been to write a practical, easy-to-read book that will teach you the latest neuroscience research on how to achieve the best brain function possible—your ultimate brain. The brain is the supercomputer that runs your life. Improving brain function enhances your ability to love, work, and learn. The principles and exercises in this book are based on years of cutting-edge neuroscience research with thousands of people who have come to the Amen Clinics, such as Bart, Angela, Marian, and John.

Over the last fifteen years the Amen Clinics have amassed the world's largest database of brain scans related to behavior. We look at the brain on a daily basis using a sophisticated study called brain SPECT imaging. We have looked at healthy brains and brains in trouble. We have looked at the brains of young children, teenagers, adults, and the elderly. We have looked at brains on medication, drug and alcohol abuse, supplements, prayer and meditation, gratitude, and a wide variety of psychological and biological treatments. At our clinics we look at, optimize, and restore the brain. This book will describe many of the lessons we have learned in the process.

THE PROGRAM

The Amen Clinic program offers a wealth of practical information on how to achieve the best brain possible. It starts by teaching you to protect your brain from injuries, toxic substances (such as alcohol and too much caffeine), and lack of sleep. It gives practical instructions on how to eat so your brain is properly nourished, and how to do mental workouts to keep your brain strong. A critical component of the program is physical exercise, which boosts blood flow and other positive nutrients to the brain. But not just any exercise will do: your exercise should get your heart rate up (helping your heart) and involve the coordination centers of the brain, as dancing and tennis do. The program teaches about the brain's need for physical affection, as well as how to rid your brain of bad thoughts that interfere with love and health. Another important part of the program deals with music. Listening to certain types of music enhances brain function; other types may have a negative impact. Ways to counteract stress are explored, as it has been recently discovered that chronic stress disrupts neural pathways and kills certain brain cells. The program concludes with ways to keep the brain healthy as you age, how to use nutritional supplements throughout life to enhance brain function, and a fifteen-day program to get started on the right path.

Come join me on one of the most important journeys of your life— a journey into the health and longevity of your brain.

PART I

NINE BRAIN-CENTERED PRINCIPLES TO CHANGE YOUR LIFE

1

YOUR BRAIN IS INVOLVED IN
EVERYTHING YOU DO

*The great sins of the world take place in the brain: but it is in the brain
that everything takes place . . . It is in the brain that the poppy is red,
that the apple is odorous, that the skylark sings, (and that we love and
hate each other).*

—Oscar Wilde

Your brain is involved in everything you do. This is the first principle of
the Amen Clinics. The sensation of waking up cuddled next to your husband's or wife's warm body is felt in the brain. The brain directs your urge to
make love and be physically close. Getting ready for the day by planning,
grooming, eating, and communicating with your husband and kids is directed by the brain. Negotiating traffic, while talking on your cell phone, is a
result of your brain giving orders. Managing your business, planning trips,
evaluating employees, running meetings, attending luncheons, and answer-
ing e-mails are all accomplished by your brain's hard work. Leaving the office
on time, playing tennis, lifting weights, and joking with your friends to un-
wind are activities spearheaded by the brain. Enjoying the sunset, helping
the kids with homework, and assisting your wife with dinner are a result of
moment-by-moment brain function. Your brain is the command and control center that runs your life.

Our work at the Amen Clinics is based on nine deceptively simple principles. Understanding these ideas will lay the foundation for making a good

brain great. These principles stem directly from the brain-imaging work that we have been doing intensely for the past fifteen years. Do not let the simplicity of these principles fool you. If you allow them to become part of your everyday life, they will change nearly everything you do in the direct service of brain health.

PRINCIPLE 1:
Your brain is involved in everything you do.

How you think, how you feel, how you act, and how well you get along with other people has to do with the moment-by-moment functioning of your brain. Most people know that the brain is the organ of behavior, but few people understand this principle at a deep emotional level. We spend more time and money on beautifying our hair, our skin, our clothes, and our homes than we do on caring for our brain. After looking at over thirty thousand brain scans, I have come to realize that how your brain works influences every part of who you are and what you do: from athletic skills to parenting, from management skills to your free time activities, from social aptitude to artistic talent, and from driving ability to the type of music you like. Look at any aspect of behavior—relationships, school, work, religion, sports—and in the middle of it all is brain function.

Let's take four common examples of behavior and look at them through the lens of this first principle: motherhood, business management, dating, and attending a sporting event.

There are many different types of mothers. There are mothers, like my own, who are outgoing, relaxed, fun-loving, upbeat, and playful. There are mothers who are more serious, who focus on their children's faults or tend to be too busy or preoccupied to play with them. There are mothers who constantly push their children to be their best and mothers who lead quietly by example. There are mothers who use guilt and nagging as the primary motivator of behavior, and mothers who cheer a child's every positive move. Ultimately, the type of mother a woman may be is determined by her brain. Mothers who are more serious tend to have higher amounts of activity in the prefrontal cortex (PFC). The prefrontal cortex is involved with goal-setting, planning, forethought, and judgment. High PFC levels are involved with goal-oriented behavior. Outgoing, playful, less serious mothers have a little less activity in this part of the brain. Guilt-driven mothers tend to have higher activity in the brain's emotional centers (limbic brain), which in turn causes them to focus on the negative, such as all of her child's faults. Few people know that the type of mother they have has everything to do with the moment-by-moment functioning of her brain.

There are in the world just as many different types of business managers as mothers, based in part on brain function. There are motivational managers and quiet managers. There are absent managers and micromanagers. There are managers who scream and yell to get their way and managers who encourage. There are managers who enjoy firing people and managers who hold on to employees much longer than they should. Managers who have high PFC activity tend to be very involved and directive; taken to an extreme, they are micromanagers. Managers with low PFC activity tend to be idea people and relatively hands-off; taken to an extreme, they are absent. A part of the brain that we will discuss in detail later on is the anterior cingulate gyrus, which runs lengthwise through the front part of the brain. It is the brain's gear shifter, allowing you to be flexible and shift between tasks. Managers who have good activity in this part of the brain tend to be flexible and are able to adapt to changes in the business climate. Managers who have excessive activity in this part of the brain tend to be rigid and inflexible. These managers tend to hold on to patterns of behavior long after they are helpful. Even though brains run businesses, few people think about the brain at work.

Our species has many varied ways to, as my eighteen-year-old daughter would say, hook up. Dating and mating are brain functions, even though the urges may feel like they come from lower in your body. There are shy people who rely on random chance to find a mate. There are outgoing people who will ask a hundred or more potential partners out on a date in search of their one true love. There are thoughtful, planning daters and those who do courtship on the spur of the moment. There are commitment-phobic daters who run at the first signs of attachment and those who commit too easily. There are people who are overwhelmed by feelings of insecurity and jealousy and those who lack sufficient caring. In the center of the dating scene is the brain. The brain allows us to pay attention to potential mates, to evaluate their suitability for us, to attach, to care, and to draw people toward us or push them away. The brain helps us evaluate honesty, fidelity, and reliability. Healthy PFC activity helps us follow through on our commitments, showing the other person that we are reliable, predictable, and likely to make a good dad or mom. Lower levels of activity in the PFC will make us more spontaneous and fun (with less forethought) but may also make us late for appointments, too pushy for early sex, and more driven by emotion. We often judge our dates based on looks, but we rarely consider their brain function. I believe this will change in the coming century. In fact, if you date my daughter for more than four months, you have to get a brain scan to determine if you can continue to see her. I'm not kidding.

There are many different types of sports fans, depending again, in part, on brain function. I watch many sports fans at the Staples Center in Los Angeles and at Angels Stadium in Anaheim, while undergoing the trials, tribulations, and joys of rooting for the Los Angeles Lakers and the Anaheim Angels. My big brother, Jim, is an intense fan. He yells at the referees and umpires when he thinks they make a mistake, and he often loudly second-guesses the coaches and managers when they play the subs. There are quiet fans who show little emotion and fans who seem as though they are going to wet their pants when the home team makes a mistake. There are forgiving fans and fans who hold grudges. There are fans who lack PFC activity and throw objects onto the court or field and fans with high PFC activity who worry the whole game through. There are fans who are rude to people who wear opposing jerseys and fans who make friends with the people around them. There are pseudofans who show up to be seen (Lakers games are always events), and fans who cry when the home team loses. There are family fans who use sporting events as a bonding mechanism, between father and son (or in my case, between father and two daughters). As the brain is involved in athletic skill, it is also involved in the type of sports fan you are.

The first principle, like all of the principles, is very simple. Your brain is involved in every aspect of your life and the person you are.

WHEN YOUR BRAIN WORKS RIGHT, YOU WORK RIGHT

WHEN YOUR BRAIN IS TROUBLED, YOU HAVE TROUBLE IN YOUR LIFE

Your brain determines your effectiveness in life. Even though this principle is simple, it is also controversial and a bit unsettling. The basic idea is that since your brain is involved in everything you do, it has to work at an optimal level in order for you to be your best self. When your brain works right, it is easier for you to be an effective parent, child, friend, lover, manager, or community activist. When your brain works right, you have full access to your true nature. On the other hand, when your brain is troubled you are more likely to struggle at work, in relationships, within yourself, and in society. When your brain is troubled, you have trouble being your best self and often act outside your own values, morals, and desires.

PRINCIPLE 2:
When your brain works right, you work right;
when your brain is troubled, it is hard to be your best self.

This principle came to me after looking at hundreds of scans on my own patients. Not only do I read scans, I also work directly with patients and families, looking into the lives of the people behind the images. Early in my imaging work, it became clear to me that the quality of brain function represented by the scans was very often associated with the quality of the decisions, outcomes, and emotional connections in the lives of my patients. In analyzing the images, I started to think about the difference between *will-driven behavior* and *brain-driven behavior*. Will-driven behavior comes from a healthy brain. It allows you to exert conscious choice over a situation to work in your own best interest. Will-driven behavior is goal directed and productive; it helps you reach the goals you have set for your life. An example would be deciding to go to medical school, then working diligently over time to make that happen, despite all of the various obstacles that get in your way.

Before I explain brain-driven behavior, I want to take a short side trip to teach you a little about the scans we do at the clinics. It will help clarify the difference between will-driven and brain-driven behaviors. The imaging study we do is called brain SPECT imaging. *SPECT* stands for "single photon emission computed tomography." It is a nuclear medicine study that uses tiny doses of radioisotopes to look at blood flow and activity patterns in the brain. SPECT scans are different from standard MRI and CAT scans, which show brain anatomy or what the brain physically looks like. SPECT scans look at function or how the brain works. SPECT results are actually very easy to read and understand. We look at areas of the brain that work well, areas that work too hard, and areas that do not work hard enough. We compare individual patient scans against a large database of both healthy and abnormal scans.

The images in this book are all three-dimensional (3D) brain images, of two kinds. The first kind is a *3D surface image,* which captures the top 45 percent of brain activity. It shows blood flow of the brain's cortical or outside surface. These images are helpful for visualizing areas of healthy blood flow and activity as well as those with diminished perfusion and activity. They assist us in looking at strokes, brain trauma, and the effects of drug abuse. A healthy 3D surface scan shows good, full, symmetrical activity across the brain's cortical surface (Images 2.1 and 2.2). A low level of activity shows up as a hole or a dent. The holes or dents usually represent not zero activity but low activity. To make these images, we ask the computer to look at the top 45 percent of brain activity; anything below that level shows up as a hole or a dent. We choose that number because it represents two standard deviations below normal, both from our own studies and from those of other scientific groups.

The second type of SPECT image we will look at is the *3D active image,* which compares average brain activity to the hottest 15 percent of activity. Such images are helpful in visualizing overactive brain areas, as seen in active

Healthy 3D Surface SPECT Images
(evaluates outside surface and underactive areas)

Image 2.1 Top-Down View

Image 2.2 Underside View

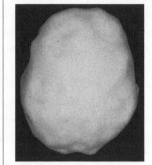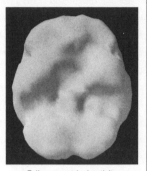

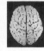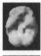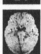

Full, symmetrical activity

Full, symmetrical activity

Healthy 3D Active SPECT Images

Image 2.3 Top-Down View
front

Image 2.4 Underside View
front

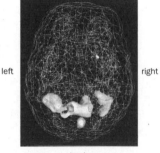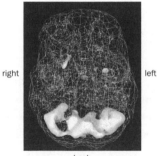

left   right   right   left

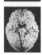

back

back

seizures, and many types of anxiety and depression, among other irregularities. A healthy 3D active scan (Images 2.3 and 2.4) reveals increased activity (shown by the light color) in the back of the brain, the cerebellum, and the visual or occipital cortex, and average activity everywhere else (shown by the background grid).

Note: These icons will be used throughout the text to help readers understand the orientation of the scans and how they differ from normal. "Image a" comprises two icons: a healthy 3D surface SPECT scan looking down at the top of the brain; the icon below it is a model of the brain viewed from the same perspective. "Image b" shows a healthy 3D surface SPECT scan viewed from below (the undersurface); the lower icon is a model of the brain from the same perspective. "Image c" shows a healthy 3D active SPECT image looking down from the top of the brain; the lower icon is a model of the brain from the same perspective. "Image d" shows a healthy 3D active SPECT image viewed from below (the undersurface); the lower icon is a model of the brain seen from the same perspective. Remember, 3D surface scans help us see underactive areas, while 3D active scans let us see overactive areas.

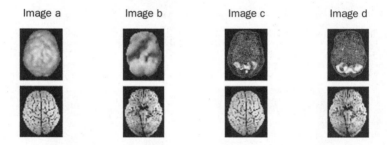

Image a   Image b   Image c   Image d

Not everyone's brain looks the same. Brains are like faces, and there is variation among them. From an aesthetic standpoint on scans, some brains are beautiful, while others may be a bit misshaped and funny-looking. Some brains are short and round, while others are long and skinny. But beautiful or not, looking at more than thirty thousand brain SPECT studies has made it clear to us that a healthy brain shows good, full, even, symmetrical activity. A healthy brain has all of its major parts intact, and they work together in a relatively harmonious fashion. Age variations are normal: the brain scans of children and teenagers reveal more activity than do those of adults. Yet even an elderly brain, if properly cared for during life, looks healthy.

Let's look at several examples of healthy and unhealthy brains. In one of the graduate courses I teach, I asked for volunteers for a healthy brain study. Christy, one of my students, came up after class very excited. "You have to scan my eighty-two-year-old grandmother, Anna," she said. "She is one of the most normal people I know. You will love her." On Christy's advice and with her grandmother's agreement, we screened her grandmother and indeed found her to be healthy and sweet; she met all the criteria for the study (no substance abuse, no brain injuries, no first-degree relatives with psychiatric illness, etc.). Anna had been married for fifty-eight years and was a loving wife, mother, and grandmother. She had a sharp, curious mind and was active in her church and community. She had solid relationships that spanned many years. Anna had one of the healthiest brains I had ever seen, out of thirty thousand (Images 2.5 and 2.6)!

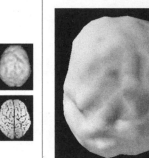
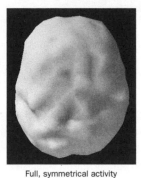
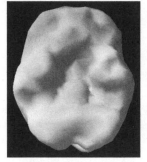
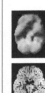

Anna's Eighty-Two-Year-Old Healthy Brain Scan

Image 2.5 Top-Down View   Image 2.6 Underside View

Full, symmetrical activity   Full, symmetrical activity

Bruce, twenty, had experienced many years of serious drug abuse, including heroin, marijuana, speed, hallucinogens, ecstasy, and pain-killers. I met him while working on a drug education video for high school students and young adults. Bruce was having problems remaining sober, he had family troubles over his drug use, and he felt ashamed about his behavior. As you can see, Anna's brain at eighty-two is much healthier than Bruce's young drug-affected brain (Image 2.7).

As we age, our brains normally get less and less active. But when an eighty-two-year-old brain looks significantly healthier than a twenty-year-old brain, then we can assume (accurately) that the twenty-year-old is in trouble.

A healthy brain, in my experience, is associated with effective, goal-directed behavior. People with healthy brains tend to make the best

Bruce's Drug-Affected Brain

Image 2.7 Top-Down View

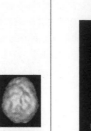

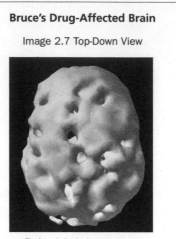

Toxic, shriveled appearance

employees, the best husbands and wives, the best parents, friends, employees, and citizens. People with troubled brains, on the other hand, tend to struggle in all areas of life. Think about Alzheimer's disease. Do you think the people who suffer from this devastating illness still have access to their full selves, to their own free will? Not possible. People with Alzheimer's disease have a serious deterioration of brain function and often behavior. My friend Leeza Gibbons, founder of Leeza's Place, a series of support centers for those afflicted with Alzheimer's disease and their families, has a mother with this devastating illness. Her mother went from being a kind, gentle, proper woman to someone who was angry, irrational, and combative. She was no longer her true self (Image 2.8).

Overactive brain activity has been associated with obsessive-compulsive disorder as well as with bipolar disorder and other conditions. Heather, a seventeen-year-old girl, was struggling with alcohol abuse when I scanned her and her brother as part of the Emmy-winning show called *The Truth About Drinking*. Even though she was only seventeen, she had already been drinking fairly heavily and was also struggling with family problems. On her scan, we saw an extremely overactive pattern of activity (Image 2.9). No wonder she drank—she was trying to settle down the pattern of overactivity in her brain.

In another example, Jimmy, a forty-five-year-old man, came to see me with post-traumatic stress disorder from being in a fire. His scan showed

An Alzheimer's Brain

Image 2.8 Top-Down View

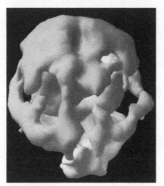

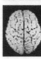

Overall severe decreased activity,
especially in back of brain

Heather's Overactive Brain

Image 2.9 Underside Active View

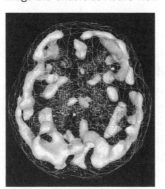

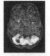

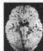

Overall marked increased activity

multiple areas of increased activity that were consistent with his anxiety, depression, and fear (Image 2.10). His emotions and emotional brain systems were working way too hard, and my job was to calm them down.

Okay, now we come back to the difference between will-driven and brain-driven behavior. Brain-driven behavior occurs when the brain hijacks

Jimmy's Overactive Brain

Image 2.10 Underside Active View

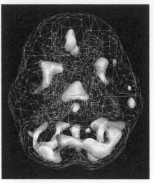
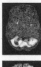
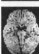

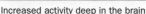

Increased activity deep in the brain

your will and causes you to act in ways that are unhelpful or even downright destructive. Patients who have obsessive-compulsive disorder (OCD), Tourette's syndrome (TS), or drug abuse are examples of people with potential brain-driven behaviors. A person who suffers from OCD has distressing repetitive thoughts and/or performs compulsive behaviors, such as excessive lock-checking or hand-washing or engaging in elaborate rituals. Even though the person knows these thoughts or behaviors are irrational, he can't just say no to them. In severe cases, the thoughts and behaviors hijack or steal the majority of his time during his waking hours. Imaging studies have revealed that patients with OCD have significant hyperactivity in the front part of the brain. They overthink (obsessions) and overact (compulsions). TS is an involuntary tic disorder, with both motor and vocal components. Even though a person with TS tries to suppress the unwanted tics, the behaviors build and build until they have to be expressed. The tics can involve facial twitches, shoulder shrugs, punching, throat-clearing, snorting, even swearing. In people with TS, scan studies have shown abnormal hyperactivity in deep-motor and emotional centers of the brain.

Drug or alcohol abuse often leads to an addiction that is out of control. Even though continued use has serious consequences, such as financial and relational disaster; even though continued use causes intense shame and self-loathing; and even though the person has tried to stop many times, she can no longer control the behavior. I once treated a thirty-two-year-old cocaine addict who was going through a divorce in large part because of his drug abuse. He had become suicidal over the prospect of losing his family. In my office, he cried about his drug use, saying it was like someone had a gun to his head—he had to use, regardless of the consequences. He had lost control over the decision of whether to use cocaine. Brain images show that sometimes drug abusers have overall low activity in the brain and use stimulants such as cocaine or methamphetamines to increase activity; sometimes they have excessive activity in the brain and are using to try to settle things down. Many lives and families have been ruined by the brain-driven behavior caused by drugs and alcohol. The addictions literally hijack the brain.

Why is this concept of will-driven versus brain-driven behavior so disturbing? It upsets the basic premise in our society that we all have the same level of free will. Isn't everyone the same? I wish it were so, but looking at tens of thousands of scans has shown me that we are not all the same. I grew up very Roman Catholic, went to Catholic schools, and was an altar boy for many years. When I was growing up, life was very clear for me. There was heaven for the good people, hell for the bad ones, and purgatory for those who weren't bad enough to go to hell but weren't good enough to get to heaven on the first try either. I believed we all had the same level of free will, a level playing field, and that on Judgment Day we would be judged based on how we behaved, how we used our talents, and of course, how we treated our mothers.

As a child, I really had no opinion on the death penalty—I just didn't give it a lot of thought. But as an adult, shortly after looking at the first brain scans I ordered, I started to get a very uncomfortable feeling. The brain function of my patients who did bad things was much worse than that of people who were living productive, healthy lives. If the brain is the organ of behavior and free will, and brain function was impaired, then obviously we all did not have the same level of free will. As I think of it, free will varies on a scale of 0 to 100. A person with a very healthy brain has nearly 100 percent free will. A patient with OCD or TS or drug addiction has significantly less, and a person with late Alzheimer's disease has virtually none. *Uh-oh,* I thought to myself, *killing people with bad brains is akin to killing sick people.* That was not the sign of an evolved society. Subsequently I have scanned more than sixty murderers and more than two hundred other convicted violent felons. The brain dysfunction I saw was often dramatic.

As I began to feel unsettled about how our society judged people, I also had personal battles to fight. When defense attorneys found out about my imaging work, they started sending me criminals to scan. We scanned violent children, teenagers, and adults, and we often found serious abnormalities in their brains. From a clinical perspective, it was very exciting work, because violent people who used to be hard to treat often got better much faster when we had the scan information to work with. We were more effective at uncovering the problems and targeting the right treatment. Now I was being asked to go into court to help explain bad behavior. Some of my colleagues, family, and prosecuting attorneys vehemently objected, and it caused quite a firestorm. Nonetheless I believed juries were entitled to the information and that as a society we needed to learn this important principle: when your brain works right, you work right, and when the brain is troubled, it is very hard to be your best self! We should be thinking about treatment rather than just punishment. The implications of this principle for society are massive. Does it mean we should screen all people who do bad things? Should we make psychiatric examinations and brain scans part of the intake process at juvenile hall? Should we rethink the death penalty?

I was recently asked to be an expert witness in a criminal case that illustrates this principle about brain function. Peter Chiesa, a sixty-two-year-old married man, was in the midst of a twelve-year feud with his next-door neighbors over trees on an easement to their property. They had litigated the feud, and even after the legal intervention they still fought about it. During those twelve years Peter's behavior became more and more irrational. He had sustained a brain injury when he fell twelve feet from the top of a haystack onto his head and lost consciousness for an undetermined period of time; he suffered a stroke; and he had coronary artery bypass surgery. This surgery has now been associated with increased risk for developing serious thinking problems and early dementia. All of these factors were likely contributing to Peter's increased paranoia and volatility. He sought psychiatric care, and his wife, twelve years younger than he, became more and more watchful over him. One day while his wife was at work, Peter woke up to the sound of a chain saw. He realized that the neighbors were cutting down the disputed tree branches.

In a rage, he called 911. "I am going to kill the motherfuckers," he shouted to the operator. "You better get someone out here immediately." He then took his .357 Magnum and confronted the two women who were violating his trees. As their two young boys watched, Peter shot and killed both women.

George Wilkinson, the psychiatrist who evaluated Peter for the defense, asked me to scan Peter's brain (Images 2.11 and 2.12). To no one's surprise, it showed severe damage, especially in the prefrontal cortex (judgment center) and the temporal lobes (associated with memory, mood stability, and aggression). The scans were used at his trial. The purpose was not to get him off—that doesn't happen, nor should it, when you kill two innocent women with their children watching—but to show the jury that Peter was not operating as a normal person with full access to his own faculties. The charges against him carried the possibility of the death penalty.

While I was on the witness stand, the prosecutor asked me, "Dr. Amen, didn't you say that Mr. Chiesa had serious problems in the prefrontal cortex, the planning part of the brain?"

"Yes, sir," I replied.

"Doesn't the fact that Mr. Chiesa called 911 ahead of time indicate good planning?" he asked sarcastically.

"No!" I said with emphasis. "Calling 911 actually indicates bad planning. What idiot would call 911 ahead of time if you planned to kill people?" I continued, "When we get upset, many people have violent thoughts, such as 'I am going to kill the motherfuckers,' but we do not call 911 or act on the bad thoughts. Good planning would have been to take a shower, make some-

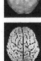
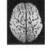
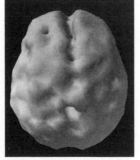
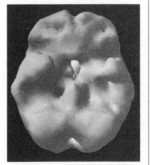

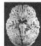

Peter's Brain (Surface Views)

Image 2.11: Top-Down View   Image 2.12: Underside View

Notice the damage in the front (top) part of Peter's brain

thing to eat, or take a walk. Good planning avoids killing people in cold blood in front of their children and helps you avoid spending the rest of your life in jail over tree branches." The prosecutor objected to my answer, but the jury heard every word. Peter was convicted of second-degree murder rather than first-degree with special circumstances and was no longer eligible for the death penalty.

Here's a more common, if less dramatic, example of brain-driven behavior. People with attention deficit disorder (ADD) are often chronically late and disorganized. Many imaging studies report that ADD is associated with low prefrontal cortex activity, the part of the brain responsible for forethought, judgment, impulse control, and organization. Jill was nearly fired from her job for chronic lateness when she came to see me. Her boss had given her the final warning. She told me that she tried to get to work on time but was late seven days out of ten. Her school history was consistent with ADD. Her teachers consistently reported problems with attention span, restlessness, poor judgment, disorganization, and underachievement. Her scans (Image 2.13) revealed low activity in her prefrontal cortex (the front third of the brain). With proper treatment and better time-management skills she was able to keep her job. It was easy for people to say she had an attitude problem, until they looked at her brain. With better brain function, Jill became a more timely, better employee.

Jill's ADD Brain (Surface View)

Image 2.13: Underside View

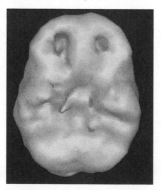

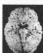

Notice the low activity in the front
(top) part of Jill's brain

When your brain works right, you work right. When your brain is troubled, it is very hard for you to be your best self. The exciting news is that with targeted treatments and appropriate interventions, such as diet, medication, supplements, exercise, and other innovative treatments, the brain can improve—even a brain as damaged as Peter's. There is much hope, but it is critical to start with the information that your brain matters and that taking care of it needs to be part of your life.

3

YOUR BRAIN IS THE MOST COMPLICATED ORGAN IN THE UNIVERSE

"The brain has the storage capacity of 6 million years of the Wall Street Journal.*"*

—Greg Iles, *Footprints of God*

Your brain is the most complex, mind-blowing organ in the universe. It weighs only about three pounds, usually around 2 percent of the body's weight. Unbelievably, given that it is the bedrock of the personality—some think even the soul—it is 80 percent water! The brain uses 20 percent of the oxygen we breathe and about 20 percent of the calories we consume. When whole-body scans are performed on people, they show the brain to be so active, compared to the rest of the body, that it looks like a small powerful heater, while everything else appears ghostlike.

The brain contains more than a hundred billion neurons (also called nerve cells or brain cells), which is about the number of stars in the Milky Way Galaxy. It also has trillions of supportive cells called glia. Each neuron is connected to other neurons by as many as forty thousand individual connections (called synapses) between cells. Multiply a hundred billion neurons times forty thousand synapses—the brain has more connections than there are stars in the universe. A piece of brain tissue the size of a grain of sand contains a hundred thousand neurons and one billion synapses, all "talking" to one another.

PRINCIPLE 3:
The human brain is the most complicated organ in the universe.

A neuron's main job is to generate an electrical signal called an action potential, which it does if it is sufficiently excited by other neurons. The action potential of a single neuron is like a lightning bolt that may stimulate other neurons. The stimulated neurons can then generate their own signals that travel to and stimulate yet other neurons to which they are connected, creating a network of neurons that perform a specific brain function. Action potentials travel down nerve cells at speeds of about sixty miles per hour. The signals can travel at these high speeds because a part of each neuron, called an axon, is wrapped in and insulated by a special substance called myelin. Like insulation surrounding an electrical wire, myelin keeps the energy focused and moving in one direction. Axons that are not insulated by myelin, either by design or disease, transmit signals ten times slower. Multiple sclerosis (MS) is called a demyelinating disease because it damages the myelin protection of neurons.

It's commonly said that we only use 10 percent of our brains. Nonsense! You may not use every neuron in your brain at the same time, but each one is important. The brain never turns off or even rests throughout your entire life. It is very active at night, especially during dreaming. We cannot take out 30 percent of your brain and have you still be you. The brain can always work at greater capacity (and we'll discuss how to get the most out of your brain), but never let anyone tell you that 90 percent is off-line.

Brain development is a fascinating construction tale, in which genes and environment collaborate to make us who we are. At some times during gestation, the fetus's brain makes 250,000 new nerve cells per minute. Babies are born with 100 billion neurons, but only a relatively small number of them are myelinated or connected. In the first decade of life, a child's brain forms trillions of connections. New research has shown that early childhood experiences do not just create a background for development and learning, they directly affect the way the brain is wired. In turn, the wiring profoundly affects our feelings, language, and thought. Experiences do not just influence a child's development; they finish the job of molding and sculpting the brain. About three-quarters of the brain develops outside the womb, in response to environment and experience. Nature and nurture always work together.

Brain development is especially rapid during the first year. Brain scans show that by twelve months a baby's brain resembles that of a normal young adult. By age three a baby's brain has formed about one thousand trillion connections—about twice as many as adult brains have. Also, the areas of the brain that develop early, such as vision, are the first areas to become myelinated (wrapped in myelin), which helps that part of the brain become more efficient. The years between ages three and ten are a time of rapid social, intellectual, emotional, and physical development. Brain activity in this age group is more than twice that of adults, and although new synapses continue to be formed throughout life, never again will the brain be able to master new skills or adapt to setbacks so easily.

At age eleven, the brain begins to prune the extra connections at a rapid rate. The circuits that remain are more specific and efficient. The brain is one of the best examples of the "use it or lose it" principle. Connections that are used repeatedly in the early years become permanent, while those that are not used are pruned.

During late adolescence and into the mid-twenties, the front third of the brain, the prefrontal cortex or executive brain, continues to develop. Even though we think of eighteen-year-olds as adults, their brains are far from finished. Myelin continues to be deposited in the PFC until age twenty-five or twenty-six, making the executive part of the brain work at a higher and more efficient level. Were you more mature at twenty-five than at eighteen? I sure was. Ironically, the car insurance industry knew about maturity and brain development long before society did. Typically, automobile insurance rates change when a driver reaches age twenty-five, because at that age drivers are more thoughtful and get into significantly fewer accidents. Their judgment centers work better.

The knowledge that brain development continues into early adulthood is critical to disseminate. Teenage and early-adult smoking, drug or alcohol abuse, and brain injuries from risky sports all have the potential to disrupt brain development, in some cases permanently.

After about twenty-five, just as we reach peak development, the brain slowly starts shrinking. Some research has suggested that the male brain shrinks faster than the female one. I think the reason is that men do more stupid things to their brains: statistically they have more problems with alcohol, they play more tackle football, and they hit more soccer balls with their heads. In college 70 percent of football players and 62 percent of soccer players get at least one concussion per year.

When it comes to the brain, *size matters*. The stegosaurus brain was about the size of a walnut. The adult human brain weighs 1,300 to 1,400 grams. The average cat brain weighs only about 30 grams. This is why human curiosity helped invent space travel and cures for cancer, while cat curiosity needs nine lives. The highly convoluted folds of gray matter on the outside surface of the brain are known as the cerebral cortex. The cerebral cortex is about two millimeters thick and has a surface area of about two and a half square feet. This is about the size of three and a half sheets of 8½-by-11-inch paper.

In order to work properly, the brain needs fuel, oxygen, and stimulation. Just like any other living thing, a brain needs fuel to grow, function, and repair itself. Glucose and oxygen run the engine powered by the brain cells. Unlike other cells in your body, glucose is the only fuel your brain knows how to use. Anything that impairs glucose delivery to brain cells is life-threatening. The brain needs oxygen to produce energy; without it, the energy powerhouses of neurons called mitochondria would not produce enough energy to keep your brain alive. Because blood delivers glucose and oxygen to the brain, nothing must get in the way of blood flow if the brain is to stay healthy. Unconsciousness will occur only eight to ten seconds after a loss of blood supply to the brain.

In addition to blood flow, the human brain is dependent on proper stimulation to grow and develop in healthy ways throughout childhood and to maintain its functioning into old age. When you stimulate neurons in the right way, you make them more efficient; they function better, and you are more likely to have an active, learning brain throughout your life. The best sources of stimulation for the brain are physical exercise, mental exercise, and social bonding, which we will discuss in greater detail later on.

If, as the New Testament says, the body is the temple of the Holy Spirit, certainly the brain is the inner sanctum.

4

YOUR BRAIN IS VERY SOFT, HOUSED IN A VERY HARD SKULL

INJURIES CAN CHANGE YOUR LIFE, AND NO ONE KNOWS ABOUT IT

You may find some of the information in this chapter scary, eye-opening, and maybe even hard to believe. But both the statistics and my experience say that it is a critical piece of the brain health puzzle and I cannot sugarcoat or gloss over it.

When the brain is alive, pulsating with activity, it is like a delicate, intricate, organized spiderweb suspended in crystal-clear fluid. The consistency of the brain has been described as being similar to soft butter, custard, tofu, or somewhere between egg whites and Jell-O. Remember, it is 85 percent water. Yet we often think of the brain as firm and rubbery, mostly because the brains dissected in anatomy labs and the ones shown on TV were fixed in formaldehyde. Your very soft brain is housed in a protective hard, thick skull. When you hold a skull in your hand and look inside, you notice that it has many ridges, some as sharp as a knife. Immediately you get the idea that an injury that rattled the soft butterlike brain could cause serious damage.

One of the most important lessons I've learned from looking at more than thirty thousand brain scans is that brain injuries, even "mild" ones without a loss of consciousness, matter more than most people, including doctors, think. Millions of people in our society have suffered significant brain injuries, yet no one knows about it. If you never look at the brain, you miss what many researchers have called the silent epidemic. Two million reported new brain injury cases occur every year, and millions of others go unnoticed.

PRINCIPLE 4:
The brain is very soft and is housed in a very hard skull. Brain injuries can change a person's whole life, and no one knows about it.

As a society, we have no respect for the physical fragility of the brain. We allow children to hit soccer balls with their heads. We allow teenage boys to take their most precious organ, put it in a hard football helmet, and slam it against other so-armed teenagers. We allow children to snowboard without helmets or ride a four-wheel vehicle in the desert, and we buy them their first motorcycles. After you read this chapter, my hope is that you will never drive without your seatbelt or allow a child to hit a soccer ball with her head.

Why are brain injuries so important? Some basic brain facts are in order here.

- Your brain is more intricate, delicate, and complicated than any computer that we can design.
- Your brain is very soft, which makes it easily bruised or damaged. When I was a little boy working in my father's grocery store, I used to see cow brains for sale in little white cups. The cow brains were so soft that they took on the shape of the cup. Human brains are the same.
- Your skull is really hard. Inside your skull there are many ridges, rough areas, and sharp bony edges.
- Your brain lives in a closed space. When you experience a blow to the head, there is no place for the brain to go, so it ends up slamming against the walls, ridges, and sharp bony edges in the skull, ripping small blood vessels, causing multiple minute bleeds and over time many areas of tiny scars.
- You do not have to lose consciousness in order to have a significant brain injury. Consciousness is controlled by structures deep in the brain. A significant injury may occur to the cortex or outside surface of the brain, sparing the brainstem and therefore causing no loss of consciousness.
- Brain injuries tend to be additive. When an injury damages a certain part of the brain, not all people have symptoms, because the brain has built-in reserves. For example, one needs to kill 30 percent of the

hippocampus (an area on the inside of the temporal lobes) before memory symptoms occur. Usually they develop vulnerabilities. The next brain injury, even if it seems minor, may wipe out the reserve, causing major problems.

- Many people forget or do not realize that they have had a serious brain injury. In our clinic we ask people five or six times whether they have had a brain or head injury. You would be amazed at how many people, after repeatedly saying no to this question, suddenly get an *aha* look on their face and say, "Why yes, I fell out of a second-story window at age seven." Or they suddenly remember they went through the windshield of a car headfirst, or had a concussion playing football or soccer, or fell down a flight of stairs.

- Not all brain injuries, even serious ones, will cause damage. The brain is buffered by clear fluid called cerebrospinal fluid (CSF). CSF helps to buffer the brain against injury. Still, damage can occur more than most people know.

One patient stands out in my memory over all others. Mark was a twenty-six-year-old man with Tourette's syndrome, a disorder that causes both motor and vocal tics. About 15 percent of people with TS have coprolalia or compulsive swearing. Mark was being treated for drug abuse and was in the middle of his hospital program when he was brought to our clinic. The third time I asked him about a head injury, he started to get irritated at me and swore, "F——— no!"

Having seen his scan (Image 4.1), I knew I had to persist. I asked if he'd ever played sports, a common question that frequently elicits forgotten head injuries.

"F——— no!" he replied, more agitated than before.

I then asked him if he had ever been in a car accident.

"F——— no!" he said once again. As his irritation with me escalated, all of a sudden he stopped, got a quizzical look on his face, and said, "Does a motorcycle accident count?"

"Tell me about it," I said.

"I was riding my motorcycle around a lake," he said, now animated and cooperative, "when all of a sudden a baby deer darted out in front of me. To miss the deer I spilled the bike on my left side. I wasn't wearing a helmet and broke my left jawbone. Do you think that counts as a head injury?"

Mark's Trauma Brain (Surface View)

Image 4.1 Underside View

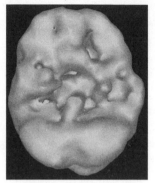

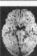

Notice the low activity on the left
side of Mark's brain

Caught up in the moment and amazed that he hadn't told me this information before, even though I had asked seven times, I answered, "F———— yes!"

A concussion or mild "traumatic brain injury" (TBI) is far more than just a bump on the head. According to the American Academy of Neurology, "There is no such thing as a minor concussion." A study from UCLA found that "the level of brain glucose use in people who suffered mild concussions was similar to that in comatose, severely brain-injured patients . . . Even mild head injuries result in major changes to the brain's metabolism and could make victims susceptible to more serious damage from a repeated blow." According to lead researcher Dr. Marvin Bergsneider, "We know that just because people are walkie-talkies—because they can walk and talk— that that's not the full story . . . Many people blow off [concussions] as being innocuous. What this study indicates in that clearly concussions can be serious."

While often there are no immediate symptoms with a concussion and nothing irregular shows up on the CT scan or the MRI, subtle changes occur. Over a period of a few weeks or even months, the individual may become tearful, angry, or irritable; have trouble thinking clearly or concentrating; or suffer from headaches, confusion, blurred vision, memory loss, or nausea. Other devastating symptoms can occur as if in slow motion. There may be personality changes, temper problems, dark thoughts, and difficulty expressing emotions or understanding others. Recovery, according to Dr. David A. Hovda, the director of the Brain Injury Research Center at UCLA, depends not only on the severity of the blow but also on how many previous concussions a person has suffered. Once a person has suffered a concussion, he or she is as much as four times more likely to sustain a second one.

Concussions can occur in many different ways. Transportation-related incidents cause the greatest number, 47 percent of all concussions. These include automobile accidents, biking accidents, snowboarding, sledding, injuries occurring while walking (such as when author Stephen King was hit by a car), or while in-line skating or skateboarding. The number of pedestrian and bicycle collisions with motor vehicles increase among school-age children. Kids unrestrained or improperly restrained in cars are at risk for traumatic brain injury as well. Inappropriate restraint devices resulted in a 3.5-fold increased risk of significant injury and a more than fourfold increased risk of significant head injury for the two-to-five-year-olds. Domestic falls account for 27 percent of the traumatic brain injuries among children. More people (of all ages) die from home falls than from home fires.

Older people, who may be unsteady on their feet, are especially prone to falls; one-third of people over sixty-five fall at least once a year. While most may worry about breaking a hip or suffering other fractures during a fall, traumatic brain injury should also be of major concern. Individuals with neurological problems such as Parkinson's disease or a prior stroke, or those suffering from the effects of multiple medications or poor eyesight due to cataracts or macular degeneration, may be most susceptible to falling. Concussions are a frequent outcome of physical abuse and one often not reported, as the individual involved may be reluctant to seek medical aid.

The American Academy of Pediatrics has warned that "on repetitive heading of soccer balls in young athletes, the bottom line is probably 'less is better.'" Heading drills, in which a child's head is knocked repeatedly, as happens with forward and defensive players, are of greater concern to pediatricians than is the occasional head-punt in a game. A pair of studies conducted in Norway and in the United States compared the mental functioning of large groups of adult soccer players to adults of similar age and circumstances who did not play soccer. Out of 106 soccer players in the Norwegian study, 81 percent had impairment of attention, concentration, memory, and judgment that ranged from mild to severe. In the U.S. study, attention and concentration deficits were significantly more common among those who "headed" the ball most often. When it comes to brain injury, football is no better than soccer. Football players are struck in the head thirty to fifty times per game and regularly endure blows similar to those experienced in car crashes, according to a Virginia Tech study that fitted players' helmets with the same kinds of sensors that trigger auto airbags.

Golf is good. Tennis is terrific. Table tennis is the world's best sport! Football, boxing, and soccer are bad for the brain! As a society, we need to seriously rethink what we allow our children to do.

WHERE IS THE BRAIN VULNERABLE?

A number of brain areas are especially vulnerable to injury (see Images 5.1 and 5.2). These include:

- The prefrontal cortex, at the front of the brain, where judgment, concentration, attention span, impulse control, organization, planning, and expressive language are centered.
- The anterior cingulate gyrus, the brain's "gear shifter," which runs deep through the front part of the brain, where damage causes people to get stuck on negative thoughts or behaviors.
- The parietal lobes, at the top back part of the brain, coordinate and interpret sensory information from the opposite side of the body; they also handle directions, construction, and advanced mathematics.
- The temporal lobes, underneath the temples and behind the eyes, which house memory, receptive language, temper control, and mood stability.
- The limbic system, deep within the brain, which can cause problems with depression, negativity, and libido.
- The occipital lobes, at the back of the brain, which can cause problems with visual processing.

Brain injuries can interrupt, delay, or alter social and intellectual development, sometimes seriously. A number of years ago I wrote a newspaper article on brain injuries. The day the article appeared in the paper, I received a call from a distraught mother. Four years earlier her sixteen-year-old son had sustained a brain injury from a bicycle accident. The front tire of his bicycle hit a curb, and he flipped over the handlebars onto the left side of his face. He was unconscious for about thirty minutes. Over the next several months his personality changed. He went from being a straight-A student and a sweet young man to being someone who had no interest in school and was easily angered and depressed. He also started frequent use of alcohol. Three years later he shot and killed himself. The mother had blamed herself for his downward spiral. No one had told her that a minor brain injury could ruin her son's life. My article helped her understand the terrible tragedy. I only wish a doctor could have diagnosed her son's brain trauma sooner so he could have been properly treated and this senseless tragedy avoided.

The good news is that brain injuries can be treated. Medication, therapy, and cognitive retraining have all been found to be helpful. We cannot prevent all injuries, so early diagnosis and proper treatment is essential. The most important strategy for us as a society is to prevent injuries by respecting the brain and stopping reckless, stupid behavior.

SOME THOUGHTS ON PREVENTION:

- Think about your brain before you do activities that might put it at risk.
- Kids must wear protective gear while playing football and hockey; do not let them hit soccer balls with their heads, and encourage them to play noncontact sports.
- Always fasten your seatbelt in a car.
- Use age-appropriate restraints in the backseat of a car when transporting children.
- Always wear a helmet when you ride a bike (even as an adult).
- Stay off motorcycles.
- Walk facing automobile traffic, not with your back toward it.
- Use a proper ladder to reach something high up rather than a chair or countertop.
- Never shake a baby or a toddler.
- Always fasten the safety belt on a high chair and a changing table.
- Use a safety gate to protect toddlers from falling down stairs.

Your brain is soft, your skull is hard. After looking at thirty thousand brain scans, I would not let my children hit a soccer ball with their heads, play tackle football, or snowboard without a helmet. I encourage my own kids to play tennis, golf, table tennis, and track. Your brain matters. Respect and protect it.

KNOW AND HEAL THE BRAIN
SYSTEMS THAT RUN YOUR LIFE

AMEN CLINIC BRAIN SYSTEM QUIZ

Whatever any man does he first must do in his mind, whose machinery is the brain. The mind can do only what the brain is equipped to do, and so man must find out what kind of brain he has before he can understand his own behavior.

—Gay Gaer Luce and Julius Segal, *Sleep*, 1966

To make a good brain great, it is important to have a basic understanding of how the brain works, including its strengths and weaknesses. This chapter will be a practical hands-on guide to doing just that. One of the basic principles of our work is that certain parts of the brain tend to do certain things, and that problems in specific areas tend to cause identifiable troubles.

PRINCIPLE 5:
**Certain brain systems are involved in specific behaviors
and cause identifiable problems when they misfire,
but these systems can be targeted and treated.**

Before I describe some of the main systems involved with behavior, take the following quiz to see where you stand. Not everyone is able to get a brain scan, so I have developed this checklist to help predict areas of strength and weakness. A word of caution is in order. Self-report quizzes have both advantages and limitations. They are quick, inexpensive, and easy to score. On the other hand, people filling them out may portray themselves in a way they want to be perceived, resulting in self-report bias. For example, some people exaggerate their experience and mark all of the symptoms as frequent, in essence saying, "I'm glad to have a real problem so that I can get help, be sick, or have an excuse for the troubles I have." Others are in total denial. They do not want to see any personal flaws, and they do not check any symptoms as problematic, in essence saying, "I'm okay. There's nothing wrong with me. Leave me alone." Not all self-report bias is intentional. People may genuinely have difficulty recognizing problems and expressing how they feel. Sometimes family members or friends are better at evaluating a loved one's level of functioning than a person evaluating himself. They may have noticed things that their loved one hasn't. No quiz of any sort should ever be used as the only assessment tool. It is simply a catalyst to make you think, ask better questions, and get more evaluation if needed.

Making a Good Brain Great Quiz
Copyright 2005 Daniel G. Amen, M.D.

Please rate yourself on each of the symptoms listed below using the following scale. If possible, to give us the most complete picture, have another person who knows you well (such as a spouse, lover, or parent) rate you as well.

0	1	2	3	4
Never	Rarely	Occasionally	Frequently	Very Frequently

OTHER   SELF

_____ ____ 1. Failure to give close attention to details; careless mistakes

_____ ____ 2. Trouble sustaining attention in routine situations (e.g., homework, chores, paperwork)

_____ ____ 3. Trouble listening

_____ ____ 4. Failure to finish things, procrastination

_____ ____ 5. Poor time organization

_____ ____ 6. Loses things

_____ ____ 7. Easily distracted

_____ ____ 8. Poor planning skills, lack of clear goals or forward thinking

_____ ____ 9. Difficulty expressing empathy for others

_____ ____ 10. Impulsiveness (saying or doing things without thinking first)

_____ ___ 11. Excessive or senseless worrying

_____ ___ 12. Upset when things do not go your way

_____ ___ 13. Upset when things are out of place

_____ ___ 14. Tendency to be oppositional or argumentative

_____ ___ 15. Tendency to have repetitive negative thoughts

_____ ___ 16. Tendency toward compulsive behaviors

_____ ___ 17. Intense dislike for change

_____ ___ 18. Tendency to hold grudges

_____ ___ 19. Needing to have things done a certain way or you become very upset

_____ ___ 20. Tendency to say no without first thinking about question

_____ ___ 21. Frequent feelings of sadness or moodiness

_____ ___ 22. Negativity

_____ ___ 23. Decreased interest in things that are usually fun or pleasurable

_____ ___ 24. Feelings of hopelessness about the future

_____ ___ 25. Feelings of worthlessness, helplessness, or powerlessness

_____ ___ 26. Feeling dissatisfied or bored

_____ ___ 27. Crying spells

_____ ___ 28. Sleep changes (too much or too little)

_____ ___ 29. Appetite changes (too much or too little)

_____ ___ 30. Chronic low self-esteem

_____ ___ 31. Frequent feelings of nervousness or anxiety

_____ ___ 32. Symptoms of heightened muscle tension (headaches, sore muscles, hand tremors)

_____ ___ 33. Tendency to predict the worst

_____ ___ 34. Conflict avoidance

_____ ___ 35. Excessive fear of being judged or scrutinized by others

_____ ___ 36. Excessive motivation, can't stop working

_____ ___ 37. Tendency to freeze in anxiety-provoking situations

_____ ___ 38. Shyness or timidity

_____ ___ 39. Sensitivity to criticism

_____ ___ 40. Fingernail-biting or skin-picking

_____ ___ 41. Trouble finding the right word

_____ ___ 42. Mood instability or changes

_____ ___ 43. Short fuse, aggression, or periods of extreme irritability

_____ _____ 44. Frequent misinterpretation of comments as negative when they are not

_____ _____ 45. Periods of panic and/or fear for no specific reason

_____ _____ 46. Visual or auditory changes, such as seeing shadows or hearing muffled sounds

_____ _____ 47. Frequent periods of déjà vu (feelings of being somewhere you have never been)

_____ _____ 48. Sensitivity or mild paranoia

_____ _____ 49. Dark thoughts, may involve suicidal or homicidal thoughts

_____ _____ 50. Periods of forgetfulness or memory problems

_____ _____ 51. Poor handwriting

_____ _____ 52. Trouble maintaining an organized work area

_____ _____ 53. Tendency to have multiple piles around the house

_____ _____ 54. Greater sensitivity to noise

_____ _____ 55. Particular sensitivity to touch or to certain clothing or tags on the clothing

_____ _____ 56. Tendency to be clumsy or accident-prone

_____ _____ 57. Trouble learning new information or routines

_____ _____ 58. Trouble keeping up in conversations

_____ _____ 59. Light sensitivity; easily bothered by glare, sunlight, headlights, or streetlights

_____ _____ 60. More sensitivity than others to the environment

ANSWER KEY

Prefrontal cortex (PFC) symptoms, questions 1–10

Anterior cingulate gyrus (ACG) symptoms, questions 11–20

Deep limbic system (DLS) symptoms, questions 21–30

Basal ganglia (BG) symptoms, questions 31–40

Temporal lobe (TL) symptoms, questions 41–50

Cerebellum (CB) symptoms, questions 51–60

Here is the probability that problems may be present in each system. How many questions did you answer with 3 or 4?

6 questions   highly probable

4 questions   probable

2 questions   may be possible

Pay particular attention to the systems for which you answered 3 or 4 to two or more questions.

Given that there are more than two thousand structures in the brain with miles of interconnections, I will by necessity oversimplify things here. The brain is divided into four main lobes or regions: frontal (forethought and judgment), temporal (memory and mood stability), parietal (sensory processing and direction sense), and occipital (visual processing) (Image 5.1). There are also important structures deep in the brain, such as the anterior cingulate gyrus (gear shifter), basal ganglia (anxiety center), and deep limbic system (emotional center), plus a very important structure at the back bottom part of the brain called the cerebellum or "little brain" (Image 5.2). A useful generalization about how the brain functions is that the back half—

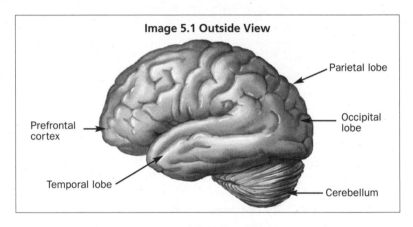

Image 5.1 Outside View

Parietal lobe

Occipital lobe

Prefrontal cortex

Temporal lobe

Cerebellum

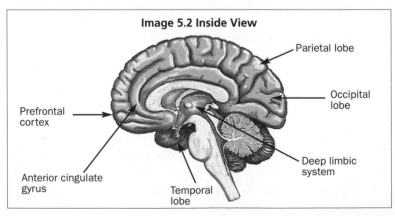

Image 5.2 Inside View

Parietal lobe

Occipital lobe

Prefrontal cortex

Deep limbic system

Anterior cingulate gyrus

Temporal lobe

the parietal, occipital, and back part of the temporal lobes—takes in and perceives the world, while the front half integrates this information, analyzes it, decides what to do, then plans and executes the decision. All of these areas are involved with your successes and struggles in life.

We'll look at the functions of six brain systems involved with work, loving, and learning, including the prefrontal cortex, anterior cingulate gyrus, deep limbic system, basal ganglia, temporal lobes, and the cerebellum. I'll briefly discuss the problems associated with each area and offer some strategies to help them heal. Never forget that with each brain system, balanced function is key.

FRONTAL AND PREFRONTAL CORTEX

The frontal lobes (the front half of the brain) are divided into three areas: the motor cortex, which controls the body's motor movements (such as walking, chewing, and moving fingers and toes); the premotor area, which is involved in planning motor movements; and the prefrontal cortex, which is involved with executive functions such as planning, forethought, judgment, organizing, impulse control, and expressing what is on your mind.

The PFC is the most evolved part of the human brain, representing 30 percent of the entire cortex. In the chimpanzee, our closest primate cousin, the PFC occupies only 11 percent; a dog's PFC is only 7 percent; and a cat's PFC, only 3.5 percent. This concept fits my cat Annabelle, who has no forethought or judgment. She lives totally in the moment and will drink out of the toilet, no matter how many times she has been told *no*. The prefrontal cortex houses our ability to learn from mistakes, make plans, and match our behavior over time to reach our goals. When the PFC works as it should, we are thoughtful, empathic, expressive, organized, and goal-oriented. The PFC is often called the executive part of the brain, like the boss at work. When it is low in activity, it is as if the boss is gone, so there is little to no supervision and nothing gets done. When the PFC works too hard, it is as if the boss is micromanaging everyone, and people are left with anxiety and worry. I call the PFC the Jiminy Cricket part of the brain. It houses our conscience and our ability to stay on track toward our goals. It is the part of the brain that, as Jiminy Cricket says in the movie *Pinocchio*, "is the still small voice that helps you decide between right and wrong."

Problems with the PFC result in a "Jiminy Cricket Deficiency Syndrome": a diminished conscience, poor judgment, impulsivity, short attention span,

PREFRONTAL CORTEX SUMMARY
(THE BOSS IN YOUR HEAD, SUPERVISING YOUR LIFE)

PFC Functions (supervision)	Low PFC Problems (lack of supervision)
Focus	Short attention span
Forethought	Lacks clear goals or forward thinking
Impulse Control	Impulsivity
Organization	Disorganization
Planning, goal-setting	Procrastination
Judgment	Poor judgment
Empathy	Lack of empathy
Emotional control	Fails to give close attention to detail
Insight	Lack of insight
Learning from mistakes	Trouble learning from mistakes
	Loses things
	Easily distracted

Diagnostic Problems Associated with Low PFC Activity

ADHD	Some types of depression
Brain trauma	Dementia, associated with bad judgment
Schizophrenia	Antisocial personality
Conduct disorders	

Diagnostic Problems Associated with High PFC Activity

Overfocused, rigid, and inflexible problems
(same as for the anterior cingulate gyrus, page 40)

Ways to Balance Low PFC

Organizational help, coaching	Intense aerobic exercise (boosts blood flow)
Goal-setting/planning exercises	Neurofeedback
Relationship counseling	Stimulating or exciting activities
Higher-protein diet	Develop a deep sense of personal meaning

Stimulating Supplements, to boost dopamine to the brain, such as L-tyrosine or SAMe

Stimulating Medications (if appropriate), such as Adderall, Dexedrine, Ritalin, Wellbutrin, Strattera, or Provigil. We generally do not give stimulants to people with schizophrenia. Obviously, any medication recommendations must be discussed with your doctor. These are just general suggestions.

disorganization, trouble learning from experience, confusion, poor time management, and lack of empathy. Low activity in this part of the brain is often due to a deficiency in the neurotransmitter dopamine; increasing it through supplements or medications is often helpful. Here is a quick summary of the PFC.

Healthy activity in the PFC is associated with conscientiousness; abnormal PFC activity is associated with inconsistency and troubled decisions. Research has established this principle as a predictor of longevity. In reviewing 194 studies Drs. T. Boggs and B. W. Roberts from the department of psychology at the University of Illinois at Urbana-Champaign found that increased death rates were associated with impulsive behaviors (a lack of conscientiousness)—tobacco use, diet and activity patterns, excessive alcohol use, violence, risky sexual behavior, risky driving, suicide, and drug use. You need a good PFC to live long and be happy!

ANTERIOR CINGULATE GYRUS (ACG)

The ACG helps you feel settled, relaxed, and flexible. It runs lengthwise through the deep parts of the frontal lobes and is the brain's major switching station. I think of it as the brain's gear shifter, greasing our behavior and allowing us to be flexible and adaptable and to change as change is needed. This part of the brain is involved in helping shift attention from thing to thing, moving from idea to idea, and seeing the options in your life. The term that best relates to the ACG is *cognitive flexibility.* When there is too much activity in the ACG, usually due to lower serotonin levels, people are unable to shift their attention and become rigid, cognitively inflexible, over-focused, anxious, and oppositional. This part of the brain influences not only shifting attention but cooperation. When the ACG works in an effective manner, it is easy to shift into cooperative modes of behavior. When it works too hard, people have difficulty shifting attention and get stuck in ineffective behavior patterns, where they may be uncooperative or difficult, stuck in their own mind-set.

The ACG has also been implicated in "future-oriented thinking," such as planning and goal-setting. When it works well, people are able to plan their future in a reasonable way. When it is underactive, people have little motivation or get-up-and-go. Damage to this part of the brain causes a condition called akinetic mutism, where people have low movement (akinetic) and little speech (mutism). When the ACG works too hard, people plan too

ANTERIOR CINGULATE GYRUS (ACG) SUMMARY
(THE BRAIN'S GEAR SHIFTER)

ACG Functions	Excessive ACG Activity Problems
Brain's gear shifter	Gets stuck on negative thoughts or behaviors
Cognitive flexibility	Worries
Cooperation	Holds grudges
Go from idea to idea	Obsessions/compulsions
See options	Inflexible, may appear selfish
Go with the flow	Oppositional/argumentative
	Upset when things do not go your way
	Upset when things are out of place
	Intense dislike for change
	Tend to say no without thinking

Diagnostic Problems Associated with Excessive ACG Activity

Obsessive compulsive disorder	Addictions
Eating disorders	Premenstrual tension syndrome, some types
Chronic pain (stuck on pain)	Post-traumatic stress disorder
Oppositional defiant disorder	Difficult temperament (need to have one's
Tourette's syndrome	own way)

Diagnostic Problems Associated with Low ACG Activity

Lowered motivation, little spontaneous movement or speech
(same as for the prefrontal cortex, page 38)

Ways to Calm Excessive ACG Activity

Neurofeedback	Intense aerobic exercise
Relationship counseling,	Lower protein/complex-carb diet
anger management	

ACG Supplements, to boost serotonin to the brain, such as 5-HTP, St. John's wort, or inositol

ACG Medications (if appropriate), SSRIs (Paxil, Zoloft, Celexa, Prozac, Luvox); Effexor; atypical antipsychotics in refractory cases, such as Risperdal, Zyprexa, or Geodon

much, worry too much about the future, and become too serious or obsessed. Difficulties in the ACG can cause a person to constantly expect negative events and feel very unsafe in the world. When the ACG is overactive, people have a tendency to get stuck or locked into negative thoughts or behaviors. They may become obsessive worriers or hold on to hurts or grudges from the past. They may also get stuck on negative behaviors or develop compulsions such as hand-washing or excessively checking locks. One patient who had ACG problems described the phenomenon as "like being on a rat's exercise wheel, where the thoughts just go over and over and over." Another patient told me, "It's like having a reset button in your head that is always on. Even though I don't want to have the thought anymore, it just keeps coming back."

The problems associated with excessive ACG activity include obsessive-compulsive disorder, eating disorders, addictive disorders, and oppositional defiant disorder. All of these disorders are associated with problems shifting attention. There are also a number of *subclinical patterns* associated with abnormalities in this part of the brain. The term *subclinical* relates to problem traits that do not reach the same level of intensity as a disorder but still cause difficulties in a person's life. Examples of these problems include worrying, holding on to hurts from the past, cognitive inflexibility, automatically saying no, and being rigid. High activity in the ACG is often due to a deficiency in the neurotransmitter serotonin, and increasing it through supplements or medications is often helpful. See page 40 for a quick summary of the ACG.

DEEP LIMBIC SYSTEM (DLS)

The DLS lies near the center of the brain. About the size of a walnut, this part of the brain is involved in setting a person's emotional tone. When the DLS is less active, the person has generally a positive, more hopeful state of mind. When it is heated up or overactive, negativity can take over. Due to this emotional shading, the DLS provides the filter through which you interpret the events of the day; it tags or colors events, depending on your emotional state of mind. The DLS, including structures called the hippocampus and amygdala, have also been reported to store highly charged emotional memories, both positive and negative. The total experience of our emotional memories is responsible, in part, for our emotional tone. Stable, positive experiences enhance how we feel. Trauma and negative experiences set our brain in a negative way.

DEEP LIMBIC SYSTEM (DLS) SUMMARY
(THE MOOD AND BONDING CENTER)

DLS Functions	Excessive DLS Activity Problems
Mood control	Depression, sadness
Charged memories	Focused on the negative, irritability
Modulates motivation	Low motivation and energy
Sets emotional tone	Negativity, blame, guilt
Appetite/sleep cycles	Poor sleep and appetite
Bonding	Social disconnections/isolation
Sense of smell	Low self-esteem
Libido	Low libido
Flight-or-fight response	Hopelessness
	Decreased interest in things that are usually fun
	Feelings of worthlessness or helplessness
	Feeling dissatisfied or bored
	Crying spells

Diagnostic Problems Associated with Excessive DLS Activity

Depression	Cyclic mood disorders
Pain syndromes	

Diagnostic Problems Associated with Low DLS Activity

Lowered motivation, decreased reactiveness, misread incoming information

Ways to Balance High DLS Activity

Biofeedback, increase left PFC activity (helps connections to DLS)
Intense aerobic exercise
Relationship counseling
Cognitive-behavioral strategies to deal with automatic negative thoughts
Balanced diet, such as described by Barry Sears in *The Zone*

DLS Supplements, such as DL phenylalanine, SAMe, L-tyrosine

DLS Medications (if appropriate), antidepressants such as Wellbutrin (bupro-prion), Effexor (venlafaxine), Norpramin (desipramine), Tofranil (imipramine), SSRIs (if ACG also present); anticonvulsants/lithium for focal increased activity or cyclic mood changes

The DLS also affects motivation and drive. It helps get you going in the morning, and it encourages you to move throughout the day. Overactivity in this area is associated with lowered motivation and drive, which is often seen in depression. The DLS controls the sleep and appetite cycles of the body and is intimately involved with bonding and social connectedness. This capacity to bond plays a significant role in the tone and quality of our moods. The DLS also directly processes the sense of smell. Because your sense of smell goes directly to the deep limbic system, it is easy to see why smells can have such a powerful impact on our feeling states.

Problems in the DLS are associated with depression, negativity, and low motivation, libido, and energy. Because sufferers feel hopeless about the outcome, they have little willpower to follow through with a task. Since the sleep and appetite centers are in the DLS, disruption can lead to changes in habits, which may mean an inclination to too much or too little of either. For example, in typical depressive episodes people have been known to lose their appetites and to have trouble sleeping despite being chronically tired. High activity in the DLS may be due to deficiencies in the neurotransmitters norepinephrine, dopamine, or serotonin; increasing these chemicals through supplements or medications may be helpful. See page 42 for a quick summary of the DLS.

BASAL GANGLIA (BG)

The basal ganglia are a set of large structures toward the center of the brain that surround the deep limbic system. The BG are involved with integrating feelings, thoughts, and movements, which is why you jump when you get excited or freeze when you are scared. The BG help to shift and smooth motor behavior. When their activity is low, as in Parkinson's disease, people can develop tremors and problems with movement (writing, walking, jumping, etc.). In our clinic we have noticed that the BG are involved with setting the body's idle or anxiety level. When the BG work too hard, people tend to struggle with anxiety and physical stress symptoms, such as headaches, intestinal problems, and muscle tension. High BG activity is also associated with conflict-avoidant behavior. Anything that reminds them of a worry (such as confronting an employee who is not doing a good job) produces anxiety, and high BG people tend to avoid it, because it makes them feel uncomfortable. People with high BG activity also have trouble relaxing and tend to overwork. When the BG are low in activity, people tend to have problems with

BASAL GANGLIA (BG) SUMMARY (THE ANXIETY CENTER)

BG Functions

Integrates feelings, thoughts, and movements

Sets body's idle

Smooths movement

Modulates motivation

Mediates pleasure

Excessive BG Activity Problems

Sets anxiety levels

Anxiety/panic

Hypervigilance

Muscle tension

Conflict avoidance

Predicts the worst

Excessive fear of being judged by others

Tendency to freeze in anxiety situations

Seems shy or timid

Bites fingernails or picks skin

Excessive motivation, can't stop working

Diagnostic Problems Associated with Excessive BG Activity

Anxiety disorders

Physical stress symptoms (headaches, stomachaches)

Workaholism

Insecurity

Diagnostic Problems Associated with Low BG Activity

Movement disorders

Low motivation

Ways to Calm High BG Activity

Body biofeedback

Hypnosis, meditation

Relaxing music

Limit caffeine/alcohol

Cognitive therapy to kill the bad thoughts

Relaxation training

Assertiveness training

BG Supplements, such as GABA or valerian root

BG Medications (if appropriate), antianxiety meds such as benzodiazepines (low dose, short time), BuSpar, antidepressants, anticonvulsants, blood pressure meds such as propranolol

motivation, attention, and moving their lives forward. In addition, the BG are involved with feelings of pleasure and ecstasy. Cocaine works in this part of the brain. High activity in the BG is often due to a deficiency in the neurotransmitter GABA; increasing it through supplements or medications is often helpful. See page 44 for a quick summary of the BG.

TEMPORAL LOBES

The temporal lobes, underneath your temples and behind your eyes, are involved with language (hearing and reading), reading social cues, short-term memory, getting memories into long-term storage, processing music, tone of voice, and mood stability. They also help with recognizing objects by sight and naming them. It is called the What Pathway in the brain, as it is involved with recognizing and naming objects and faces. In addition, the temporal lobes, especially on the right side, have been implicated in spiritual experience and insight. Experiments that stimulate the right temporal lobe have demonstrated increased religious or spiritual experiences, such as feeling God's presence.

The hippocampus, situated on the inside aspect of the temporal lobes, encodes new information and stores it for up to several weeks. When the hippocampus is damaged, you can neither store new experiences nor retrieve experiences learned within the past several weeks. The hippocampus is one of the first areas damaged by Alzheimer's disease.

In front of the hippocampus on the inside of the temporal lobe is an almond-shaped structure called the amygdala. The amygdala coordinates your emotional responses. Strong emotions can improve the encoding process of hippocampal neurons and make it easier to retrieve the experience. This is useful because it allows you to more easily remember events that were "emotionally stimulating," such as being mugged, having good sex, or recalling a fascinating fact you recently heard. I remember a taxi ride last year from Manhattan to JFK Airport like it was yesterday. I even remember the cab number, 4118. A year later. The cab driver had very irritating music on, talked loudly on his cell phone, paid little attention to the road, and nearly got us into two accidents. My emotional response to this terrible ride got his cab number stuck in my head. By emphasizing the memory of certain experiences over others, the amygdala allows you to respond more appropriately and quickly in the future—being able to recognize a potential mugger

TEMPORAL LOBES (TLS) SUMMARY (MEMORY AND MOOD STABILITY)

TL Functions	TL Problems
Understand/use language	Memory problems
Auditory learning	Auditory and visual processing problems
Retrieval of words	Trouble finding the right word
Emotional stability	Mood instability
Facilitating long memory	Anxiety for little or no reason
Reading (left side)	Headaches or abdominal pain, hard to diagnose
Read faces	Trouble reading facial expressions or social cues
Read social cues (right side)	Dark, evil, awful, or hopeless thoughts
Verbal intonation	Aggression, toward self or others
Rhythm, music	Learning problems
Visual learning	Illusions (shadows, visual or auditory distortions)
Spiritual experience	Overfocused on religious ideas

Diagnostic Problems Associated with Poor TL Activity

Head injury	Dissociation
Anxiety	Temporal epilepsy
Amnesia	Serious depression with dark or suicidal thoughts
Left side—aggression, dyslexia	Right side—trouble with social cues

Diagnostic Problems Associated with High TL Activity

Epilepsy
Religiosity
Increased intuition or sensory perception
Same interventions as low TL activity

Ways to Balance the TLs

Biofeedback to stabilize TL function	Relationship counseling
Anger management	Music therapy
Increased protein diet	

For memory problems (options to consider)

- Both physical and mental exercise
- Omega-3 fatty acids, alpha-lipoic acid, vitamin E, and vitamin C as antioxidants, phosphatidalserine, ginkgo biloba, low-dose ibuprofen (see Chapter 20)

TL Supplements, such as GABA or valerian to calm TLs if needed

TL Medications (if appropriate), antiseizure medications for mood instability and temper problems, such as Depakote, Neurontin, Gabitril, and Lamictal; memory-enhancing medications for more serious memory problems, such as Namenda, Aricept, Exelon, or Reminyl

or dangerous cab driver ahead of time may save your life. When the amygdala functions appropriately, we tend to react to the world in a logical, thoughtful way. When it is overactive, our responses may be exaggerated for the situation. When the amygdala is underactive, we fail to read situations accurately, and our response may not match what has happened. For example, if you laugh upon hearing from your wife that her best friend died, your amygdala may not be working properly.

Trouble in the temporal lobes leads to both short- and long-term memory problems, reading difficulties, trouble finding the right words in conversation, trouble reading social cues, mood instability, and sometimes religious or moral preoccupation or perhaps a lack of spiritual sensitivity. The temporal lobes, especially on the left side, have been associated with temper problems. Abnormal (high or low) activity in this part of the brain is often due to a deficiency in the neurotransmitter GABA, and balancing it through supplements or medications is often helpful. See page 46 for a quick summary of the TLS.

CEREBELLUM

The cerebellum, at the back bottom part of the brain, is called the little brain. Even though it represents only 10 percent of the brain's volume, it houses 50 percent of the brain's neurons. It has long been known that the cerebellum is involved with motor coordination, posture, and how we walk. Only recently has it become clear that the cerebellum is also involved with processing speed, like clock speed on a computer, which may be the reason it has so many neurons. It is also involved with thought coordination, or how quickly you can make cognitive and emotional adjustments. The cerebellum helps you quickly make physical adjustments, such as while you are playing a sport, and it helps you make emotional adjustments in stressful or novel situations. When there are problems in the cerebellum, people tend not only to struggle with physical coordination but also to get confused easily. Our research has found that low cerebellar activity is also associated with poor handwriting (coordination), problems maintaining an organized work area, being sensitive to light, noise, touch, or clothing (such as tags), and being clumsy or accident-prone. The cerebellum has been found to be low in activity in people with autism, attention deficit disorders, and learning disabilities.

Given that the cerebellum is the major coordination center in the brain, coordination exercises, such as sports and music, are some of the major

CEREBELLUM (CB) SUMMARY (COORDINATION AND PROCESSING SPEED)

CB Functions

Motor control
Posture, gait
Executive function, connects to PFC
Speed of cognitive integration
   (like clock speed of computer)

Low CB Activity Problems

Walking/coordination problems
Slowed thinking
Slowed speech
Impulsivity
Trouble learning routines
Poor handwriting
Trouble maintaining an organized work area
Multiple piles around the house
Greater sensitivity to noise than others
Greater sensitivity to touch
Sensitivity to certain clothing or tags on
   clothing
Clumsiness or accident-prone
Trouble learning new information or routines
Trouble keeping up in conversations
Light sensitivity

Diagnostic Problems Associated with Poor CB Activity

Trauma
Autism, Asperger's
Developmental coordination
   disorder

Alcohol abuse
Some forms of ADD
Sensory motor integration problems

Diagnostic Problems Associated with High CB Activity

unknown

Ways to Balance Low CB Activity

Prevention of brain injury
Occupational therapy
Interactive metronome

Stop alcohol use or other toxic exposure
Hyperbaric oxygen therapy
Other coordination exercises

CB Supplements unknown

CB Medications unknown

strategies to keep the brain tuned to work at its best. At this point there is uncertainty about the neurotransmitter deficiency in this part of the brain, so we do not know what supplements or medications may be helpful. See page 48 for a quick summary of the CB.

By spending time on these systems, my hope is to bring you and your brain closer. Obviously, the brain is more detailed and technical than I have described here, but having a sense of the systems that run your life will help you know your strengths and the areas that need more attention.

ONE SIZE DOES NOT FIT EVERYONE

MOST PROBLEMS (SUCH AS ADD, ANXIETY, AND DEPRESSION) ARE NOT SINGLE OR SIMPLE DISORDERS

Why would a doctor *never* give a patient a diagnosis of chest pain? Because it is a symptom, it is too broad, and it has far too many causes to be considered a diagnosis or a single entity. What can cause chest pain? Many problems, such as grief, panic attacks, hyperthyroidism, pneumonia, lung cancer, toxic exposure, a heart attack, abnormal heart rhythm, heart infection, rib injuries, indigestion, gastric reflux esophagitis, gallbladder stones, liver disease, kidney disease, and pancreatic cancer. Chest pain has many different possible causes and many possible treatments.

In the same way, what can cause depression? Again, many different problems, such as grief, loss, chronic stress, a brain injury, stroke, toxic exposure, substance abuse, hypothyroidism, post-pneumonia or heart attack depression syndrome, anemia, cancer treatments, liver disease, kidney disease, and pancreatic cancer. Depression can be caused by low activity in the brain or by overall increased activity. It can be caused by increased anterior cingulate hyperactivity (the worried sort of depression), or by increased deep limbic activity (the sad, hopeless kind of depression), or by a combination of these plus still other problems. There are many different types of depression.

How does chest pain relate to ADD, anxiety, or depression? All of these problems are symptom clusters, not causes. Many physicians and patients view these common problems as single or simple disorders, and they often have the idea that one treatment fits everyone with a certain disorder. So if you get a diagnosis of ADD, you are likely to be prescribed a stimulant medication, such as Ritalin or Adderall; if you get a diagnosis of anxiety, you are likely to be prescribed an antianxiety medication such as Xanax; if you get a diagnosis of depression, your doctor is likely to prescribe an antidepressant such as Prozac or Lexapro.

This simplistic approach to psychiatric diagnosis and treatment is a major reason that most psychiatric medications are controversial. People rarely get emotional over stomach medications, or medicines for diabetes, cancer, heart problems, or itching. But mention Ritalin or Prozac at a party, and nearly everyone has an opinion on whether it is good, bad, overprescribed, or the cause of the loss of the soul in America. This wide variety of responses and opinions is the direct result of the extreme ranges of success and failure credited to psychiatric medications.

PRINCIPLE 6:
Most problems (such as ADD, anxiety, and depression) are not single or simple disorders. One size does not fit everyone; people need an individualized approach to optimizing their brain and their life.

Principle 6 confuses some of our critics and infuriates others, but in our experience with thousands of patients, it is absolutely true. If you treat all patients with the same group of symptoms the same way, you will make some people better and a lot of people worse. In our experience, attention deficit disorder is not one illness but rather at least six different sets of problems, and if doctors immediately turn to stimulant medications for everyone who has ADD, they make four of the six types worse. Anxiety and depression are not separate homogeneous problems, but rather a combination of overlapping issues with at least seven different subtypes. While Prozac-like medications may work perfectly for some, giving all people with depression the same type of drug invites treatment failures and in some cases may cause suicide or homicide attempts. There are many different types and causes of schizophrenia, autism, and bipolar disorder. Likewise, all alcoholics are not the same, and one treatment does not work for every alcoholic. Most people who suffer from emotional or behavior problems do not neatly fit into discrete categories. Each person needs an individualized treatment plan based on the problems in his or her own specific brain. This is one of the bedrock principles of our work.

Doctors should be treating not symptoms, but rather the underlying brain problems that are causing the difficulties. When a doctor gives a patient a diagnosis of ADD, anxiety, or depression, it is like giving someone a diagnosis of chest pain. It does not honor the underlying diversity of brain issues in these problems and leads to oversimplified treatments, making many people worse and adding to the negative debate about psychiatric treatments.

The idea that "one treatment fits everyone" just doesn't fit clinical experience. How did it evolve? Many professionals put entirely too much stock in a document called the *Diagnostic and Statistical Manual* (*DSM*). With the publication of the *DSM* by the American Psychiatric Association in the 1950s, psychiatrists began a process of describing discrete psychiatric syndromes, such as schizophrenia, bipolar disorder, major depression, and obsessive-compulsive disorder. The manual, and its four subsequent revisions, attempted to bring standardization to psychiatric diagnoses so that researchers and clinicians would have a common language to study these problems. At the time it was a giant step forward from the jumbled way that psychiatric patients had previously been described.

The *DSM* was never meant to be the last word, but a continual work in progress. Unfortunately, it has now become a larger-than-life document that is often referred to as the bible of psychiatry. The *DSM* is used in court, by insurance companies, in teaching programs, by doctors making diagnoses, and by imaging researchers. The fatal flaw in the *DSM* is that on the surface it describes many psychiatric illnesses, such as depression and ADD, as homogeneous disorders. If you meet six out of nine criteria for major depression, then you have major depression and should be treated with an antidepressant. If you meet six out of nine criteria for inattention and six out of nine criteria for hyperactivity or impulsivity, then you have ADD and should be treated with a stimulant medication. Applying these medications, unfortunately, makes many patients worse.

Compounding the problem is the fact that 85 percent of psychiatric medications are prescribed by nonpsychiatric physicians. They are prescribed by pediatricians, family practice doctors, internists, cardiologists, orthopedists, and gynecologists. The lack of in-depth training among these physicians leads to an overly simplistic approach to diagnosis and treatment, ultimately wreaking havoc in many people's lives.

In 2004 I was a guest on the *Ricki Lake Show*. The subject of the show was the controversy about using psychiatric medications in children. The show's producer had read my book *Healing ADD*, and told me I would be a voice of reason. When I arrived at the studio, I got the feeling that something was wrong. They separated all of the guests in different dressing rooms so that we wouldn't talk to one another ahead of time. Why the secrecy? I wondered. They didn't tell me they had brought in another doctor who was totally against ever using medication in children. They were setting up conflict and tension, a common element in the show. As I watched the program unfold, my discomfort grew. They had several guests who had been helped by medication, but many more who had been hurt by it. It seemed that Ricki and the audience were becoming ever more frenzied against the use of psychiatric medicine in children, as if it were a political issue rather than a medical issue.

Then in the segment before I was to come on, a couple appeared onstage by themselves. They were the parents of a ten-year-old girl who had been diagnosed with ADD. She had minor learning problems in school; a teacher had thought she might have attentional problems and recommended an evaluation. The doctor who saw her agreed she had problems and put the little girl on three different antidepressants. The last one was called desipramine, the use of which had been considered controversial in children since 1991 because of four reported deaths in children taking it. Most child psychiatrists, myself included, had stopped using it for children over a decade ago. When I heard desipramine mentioned on a show that was clearly hostile to medicine, I knew that the medicine had killed the little girl. It was gut-wrenching to watch the parents tearfully describe how the doctor kept raising the dose, until one day the child started to have seizures and then died in the mother's arms. If I was supposed to be the voice of reason, what words could I possibly say to bring understanding and healing to traumatized parents and a tearful, angry audience shocked with disbelief? None seemed reasonable.

Then I found myself on the stage, with a family doctor who was opposed to medication, the parents of the deceased girl, and a hostile audience. As is my tendency in these situations, I prayed for wisdom. I started by saying that medicine is not the enemy, that it helps millions of people. The *wrong* medicine is the enemy. Using a "one treatment fits everyone" approach can cause serious problems. I said I was deeply sorry and disturbed by the loss of the little girl, especially when there were safer alternatives. The audience seemed to settle down, but in a blur the show was over, and I was taken off to JFK Airport for the trip home. When will we learn, I wondered, that people are different and need individualized treatment programs, based on what is happening in their own brains? When will we learn to use the safest alternatives before going to stronger and riskier ones?

The Amen Clinics use a brain system approach for diagnosing and treating problems. We believe that problems such as ADD, anxiety, and depression are overall categories and that effective treatment takes into account individual variations within each type. For example, patients with ADD have common symptoms that usually relate to the prefrontal cortex, such as short attention span, distractibility, disorganization, procrastination, and poor internal supervision. To treat ADD properly, it is critical to understand the complexity of ADD and the brain systems underlying each of its six subtypes. In addition, we know that there are many ways, in addition to medicine, to help balance the brain. It is our job to inform people about what they have and give them different treatment options so they can decide what is best for them. You can see my books *Healing ADD* and *Healing Anxiety and Depression* (written with psychiatrist Lisa Routh) to get a detailed explanation of the subtypes of these disorders.

One treatment does not fit everyone. We are all different and have different needs. Individualizing interventions for you and for your specific brain is important to making a good brain great! Here is a brief example of the power of this principle. The following letter, written by the father of one of my patients, is addressed to some parents who were considering bringing their child to one of our clinics (Images 6.1 and 6.2).

Twelve-Year-Old Girl

Image 6.1 Underside Active View   Image 6.2 Underside Active View

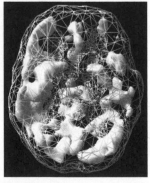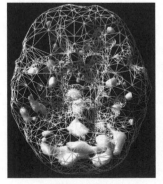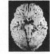

Overall, severe increased activity   Normalized activity

Dear D,

Just to give you a sense of "comfort" here . . . this is our story. My twelve-year-old had very serious behavioral issues . . . uncontrollable fits, etc., etc. She was more work than our other four kids put together . . . and had her mother and me climbing the walls as well as losing our tempers. Our pediatrician diagnosed ADD . . . and prescribed certain drugs that just made things worse. We went to Dr. Amen after a recommendation by a close friend, who is a superior court judge. After Dr. Amen's diagnosis (ring of fire) he was able to take my daughter off the drugs and on to vitamins . . . The change in behavior has been no less than a miracle . . . e.g., my daughter no longer gets STUCK and in a rage at her mother or myself.

Our pediatrician, who also recommended Dr. Amen, told us that he was about five years ahead of his time. This process certainly helped her mother and I understand (and appreciate) our daughter. We had come to the point (and even threatened several times) of sending her to a boarding school. She was having a major negative impact (with language) on our four-year-old and tormenting our three teenagers constantly. It was making our home unlivable.

D, our daughter is now my most charismatic, enjoyable, and entrepreneurial kid . . . a TRUE JEWEL. She will break all the boundaries. But now we know how or have another tool to help discipline her gifts . . . a good part being proper nutrition.

Sincerely,

C.

HOW DO YOU KNOW
UNLESS YOU LOOK?

NEW KNOWLEDGE FROM IMAGING

"The brain science of my time is not up to the task of explaining pa-tients' symptoms."
　—Sigmund Freud, "The Project for a Scientific Psychology" (1895)

"Brain imaging . . . is the future of psychiatry."
　—Steven Hyman, *Scientific American* (2003)

"He who joyfully marches to music in rank and file has already earned my contempt. He has been given a large brain by mistake, since for him the spinal cord would fully suffice."
　—Albert Einstein

In the late 1800s neurologist Sigmund Freud became obsessed with con-structing a model of the mind based on brain science. At a pivotal time in his career, in 1885, he studied with one of the founding fathers of neurology, Jean-Martin Charcot, at the Sâlpetrière Hospital in Paris. Charcot, the world's first neuropsychiatrist, understood that the mind and brain work to-gether and used hypnosis to treat patients with hysterical symptoms. After spending several months with Charcot and then treating patients in his own practice in Vienna, Freud came to believe, as his mentor had done, that hidden mental processes exert powerful effects on the conscious mind and physical brain. He postulated that hysteria (physical symptoms without a clear physical cause, such as hysterical blindness), and problems like it, resulted not from faking illness but rather from subtle changes in the brain. Try as he did to prove this connection, Freud remained frustrated that he lacked the tools to visualize and understand emotional problems and the brain. In 1895 in "The Project for a Scientific Psychology," Freud finally seemed to give up his quest when he wrote, "The brain science of my time is not up to the task of explaining patients' symptoms." Freud went on to develop psychoanalysis, which used language, emotion, relationships—and not the brain—in the healing process. He knew that one day neuroscience and psychology would be back together. His ideas were just too early to become a reality.

Over 110 years ago Freud was on to something important, but he did not have the tools to see the connection between the mind and the brain. A great deal of wonderful scientific work has been done since that time. Finally, we are now on the verge of fusing neuroscience and psychology. But today as in Freud's time, new ideas take time to be accepted.

One of the tools that have been seminal in bringing about Freud's dream is the use of functional brain imaging to understand thoughts, feelings, and behavior. With the newer imaging modalities, we can actually see what is happening in the brain while people are dreaming, thinking, obsessing, gambling, focusing, drinking alcohol or using drugs, fantasizing, and feeling sad or mad. At the Amen Clinics we have scanned young children with autism and drug exposure; children with ADD and learning disabilities; bipolar teenagers and adults; suicidal and homicidal patients; marital couples in trouble; drug, sex, and gambling addicts; pedophiles and arsonists; and almost any thought, feeling, or behavioral problem you can imagine. Twenty-eight thousand scans later, we agree with Freud: there is a huge connection between the mind and the brain. But how would you know unless you looked?

We use imaging technology to help us make difficult brains better and good brains great, because it allows us to obtain a baseline to evaluate brain health. Like whole-body scans, fast coronary artery CT scans, and fractionated cholesterol levels, brain imaging is now at the point where we can specifically see how the brain works and make targeted interventions to help it. We can see who needs help and who doesn't. Imaging allows us to see if your brain is working too hard in certain areas or not hard enough. It allows us to visualize if your brain has been hurt, traumatized, or exposed to toxic chemicals. It allows us to give people targeted help and then do follow-up scans to see if we are making the progress we want.

One of the most gratifying compliments that I have received in my career came when the chairman of the department of psychiatry at the University of California, Irvine, introduced me at a faculty retreat saying, "If Freud were alive today, he would be doing the imaging work that Dan is doing at his clinics."

PRINCIPLE 7:
Imaging the brain is essential to knowing how to help it. Imaging helps physicians be more effective, increases patient compliance, and decreases stigma. Imaging helps give direction on how to make a good brain great!

Why are psychiatrists the only medical specialists who never look at the organ they treat? For the past fifteen years I have encouraged psychiatrists to avail themselves of this new technology. Freud would have used it. Why not the modern psychiatrist? Unfortunately, the odds are that even if a patient has a serious problem with feelings (depression), thoughts (intrusive frightening ones), or behavior (aggressive or self-destructive), the treating physician will still not order a brain scan as part of the evaluation process. You can try to kill yourself in most cities of the world, and virtually no psychiatrist will look at your brain. You can kill seven people, and most prosecutors will try to keep brain-imaging science out of court. Doctors prescribe psychotherapy or powerful combinations of medications without ever looking at how an individual patient's brain works. When it comes to behavior, learning, and emotional problems, doctors prescribe treatments in the dark. The lack of brain imaging, in my opinion, has kept psychiatry lagging behind medicine's other specialties, decreasing its effectiveness with patients, and reinforcing the stigma that surrounds people who struggle with mood, learning, or behavior problems. It is time to work toward using imaging on a daily basis to look at people who struggle, and also at people who want to be better than they are.

Can you imagine the outcry that would erupt if other medical specialties acted without looking? If orthopedic doctors set broken bones without X-rays? If cardiologists diagnosed coronary artery blockages without doing angiograms or fast CT scans? Or if internists diagnosed pneumonia without ordering chest X-rays or doing sputum cultures? Yet the state of the art in psychiatry, even at the end of the first decade of the twenty-first century, is to refuse to look at the organ it treats. We diagnose and treat patients based upon symptom clusters, not upon underling brain dysfunction.

I am trained as a psychiatrist with psychoanalytic roots. I also have a specialty in children, teenagers, families, and brain imaging. In the early 1970s, before college, medical school, and my psychiatric training at the Walter Reed Army Medical Center in Washington, D.C., I was an infantry medic for the U.S. Army's Third Armored Division, stationed near Frankfurt, Germany. My specialty was as an X-ray technician. I spent most of my days taking pictures of body parts. Among other things, I took pictures of bones, lungs, abdomens, kidneys, and skulls. When I entered medical school in 1978, I was used to looking at troubled organs and using imaging in many different parts of medicine, including preventive medicine, with procedures such as chest X-rays and mammograms.

One of the most influential experiences in my professional life came when I was a third-year medical student. I was doing a pediatric rotation at St. John's Hospital in Tulsa, Oklahoma, when I met a baby boy and his worried mother. Luke was ten weeks old when his mother brought him to the hospital because he appeared to be floppy. He had little muscle tone and could not hold his head up, which was not normal at that age. The neurologist who examined the baby while I looked on was certain that Luke had been exposed to raw honey containing a certain toxic material called botulinin. The doctor said we just had to wait things out and the baby would be okay. I asked the doctor why he wouldn't order a brain scan to rule out other problems, such as a brain tumor, which was a potential cause of floppy baby syndrome. The neurologist became very irritated with me and said he was going to teach me not to order too many tests and waste money. Clinical history, he said, is the most important part of the examination. The whole incident made me very uncomfortable. How did he know without looking? I wondered. The baby continued to get worse. The neurologist dug in his heels. Finally one night on call I was urgently paged to the baby's room. It was clear that Luke had just had a stroke. He was paralyzed on one side and appeared to be blind. When we took him to X-ray, his brain scan revealed that he had a brain tumor that had just caused a stroke in the back part of his brain, resulting in permanent blindness. Luke's mother was devastated. I was sad and furious beyond words. How can you know unless you look?

This experience, along with many others, inspired me to become deeply involved in brain-imaging technology. There are so many different causes of behavior, learning, and emotional problems that I think it is unconscionable for physicians not to look at the brain, the organ of behavior, learning, and emotion.

Many people ask me why psychiatrists don't look at brain function. Frankly, the real answer is beyond my comprehension. I can't fathom why psychiatrists wouldn't want more information that helps them ask better questions and make better decisions for patients. Nonetheless, here are some potential candidate reasons.

- Doctors do not do what they are not trained to do. Imaging is usually not a part of psychiatric training programs. UC Irvine is one of the only places in the world where psychiatric residents get an in-depth education in using imaging for mental health problems.
- Imaging is not a part of psychiatric tradition. (We haven't done it in the past.)
- Most psychiatrists do not know how to look at brain scans, even when they are done, and do not know what they mean.
- Most psychiatrists do not know what to do with the information from brain scans.
- There is a perception among psychiatrists that in our age of managed care it is hard to get brain-imaging studies approved by insurance companies.
- Most psychiatrists still believe that brain-imaging tools are experimental.

It is time for psychiatrists to shed these mistaken beliefs and learn about imaging. The brain is the organ of behavior, and imaging technology can be helpful and vital to people today. As Steven Hyman, former president of Harvard University, wrote in *Scientific American* magazine in 2003, brain imaging and genetics are part of the future of psychiatry. I have argued for fifteen years that the future is now. Harold Bursztajn, director of Harvard's Psychiatry and the Law program, says that brain imaging helps physicians ask better questions. The next generation of mental health professionals is in for a wild ride, as neuroscience and psychology come back together.

The Society of Nuclear Medicine, one of the professional groups that oversee functional brain imaging, advises that there are four standard reasons to order brain SPECT studies: to evaluate suspected brain trauma, to evaluate patients with suspected dementia or cognitive decline, to evaluate seizure activity before surgery to help decide where to operate, and to detect and evaluate blood-vessel disease in the brain. The society's guidelines also say that many additional indications appear promising. At the Amen Clinics, because of our experience, we have added these further reasons to get a scan: to evaluate violence, suicidal behavior, substance abuse, subtyping ADD, anxiety and depression, and complex or resistant psychiatric problems, and to evaluate brain health for determining appropriate prevention strategies.

Imaging is a critical component of brain health and part of the future of psychiatry. Shortly after my book *Healing the Hardware of the Soul* hit bookstores in 2002, I received a very kind letter from a psychiatrist in Berkeley, who wrote,

> "All truth goes through three stages.
> First, it is ridiculed,
> Second, it is vehemently denied, and
> Third, it is accepted as self-evident."

Routine brain imaging is currently between steps two and three—some passionately deny its usefulness, while others are ordering studies. More than a thousand physicians and mental health professionals have sent patients for scans. In the next decade, imaging will become a routine part of what we do. In the Appendix you will find a more thorough discussion of brain SPECT imaging, when and why to order a scan, and common questions and answers about the technology. I realize that not everyone who needs a scan will be able to get one; the quiz in Chapter 5 will help people to get the help they need.

How do you know unless you look?

YES, YOU CAN CHANGE YOUR BRAIN AND CHANGE YOUR LIFE!

"Everyone thinks of changing the world, but no one thinks of changing himself [or his brain]."

—Leo Tolstoy

The most exciting concept in this book, and in our work at the Amen Clinics, is that the brain can change. You are not necessarily stuck with the brain you have. You can make it better! Like your body, you can start working today to increase its circulation, growth, connections, and efficiency. You can enhance your brain, your temperament, and your personality, as well as your ability to love and connect with others.

At the Amen Clinics we have performed hundreds of before-and-after SPECT scans with a wide variety of interventions, such as medication, meditation, psychotherapy, supplements, and dietary interventions. When you do the right things for the brain, you enhance it. When you do the wrong things for the brain, you make it worse. And we can prove it.

PRINCIPLE 8:
You can change your brain and change your life.

Our imaging work and the work of many other scientists have shown that many things can change the brain in a negative way, such as drug abuse, smoking, too much caffeine, head trauma, working in a toxic environment, too much stress, a lack of exercise, poor diet, a traumatic experience, negative thoughts, infection, allergic reaction, cancer treatment, coronary bypass surgery, a lack of education, and many more. The opposite is also true: you can change your brain in a positive way. Part II of this book is dedicated to helping you achieve the best brain possible, to enhance it, optimize it, and literally make it work at peak efficiency.

The first step to achieving this goal is to believe that you can change the brain. Once you develop this belief, you can put a program in place to make it happen. In this chapter I will give you four stories from my recent practice to illustrate the possibility of changing brains and changing people's lives.

JACK CAN STAY HOME

Twelve-year-old Jack was brought to my clinic by his parents. He was struggling in school, had severe temper problems, and had alienated his brothers, his sisters, and the kids in the neighborhood. His parents brought him to therapists, but he refused to get out of the car to talk to them. His pediatrician put him on four different medications, without much success. He would often spit out the medicine in front of his mother. Life was a daily battle, and Mom wanted to run away from home. They had even started the paperwork to send him away to a therapeutic boarding school—when they heard me lecture at a local church. When I met Jack, I could see that a sweet boy resided somewhere hidden inside, even though he cursed at me throughout our first meeting. His SPECT scans showed severe overall increased activity throughout his brain (Images 8.1 and 8.2). It is a pattern we call the ring of fire, because the brain looks as if it is hot or overactive throughout the cortex. For the first time since Jack's parents had begun dragging him to mental health professionals, Jack paid attention to his doctor. He asked questions about the scan and wanted to learn more about his brain. Willingly, he took the supplements and fish oil I prescribed, he worked with me to get better control over his temper, and he started to do better in school, at home, and with his friends. Four months after we began treatment, I ordered a follow-up scan on Jack. His brain, as evidenced by his loving behavior, had dramatically settled down. By changing or balancing his brain, I was able to change his life.

Jack's Brain

Image 8.1 Before Treatment   Image 8.2 After Treatment

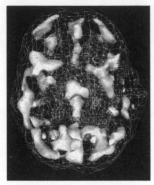
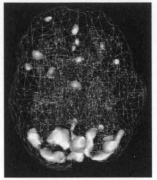
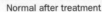

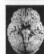

Overall increased activity,   Normal after treatment
"ring of fire" pattern

STEVEN AND THE SANTA MONICA FARMERS' MARKET DISASTER

On July 16, 2003, Steven, a thirty-three-year-old bicycle repair mechanic working in Santa Monica, California, insisted on taking an early lunch. He was not sure why he needed to go to the downtown farmers' market, but he felt drawn to it. While he was walking, eighty-seven-year-old George Russell Weller lost control of his 1992 Buick LeSabre and barreled through the three-block-long farmers market. Bodies were flying, people were screaming, and Weller's car was headed straight for Steven. Steven knew he would be hit. He later said, "I thought he was going to run over my legs . . . I thought I would lose my legs." At the last possible moment, Steven was able to jump out of the way. Then all hell broke lose. Ten people were killed, and more than fifty were injured. Steven, who had been a military tank commander in the first Gulf War, used the medical skills he had learned to help save others. Still, a woman died in his arms.

Traumatized, Steven went back to work. But for months he couldn't sleep and couldn't stop shaking. By chance—or fate, if you believe in such things—Linda Alvarez, one of the anchors at CBS News in Los Angeles, took her bicycle to Steven's shop. Shortly after the disaster, Linda and Steven talked about it in a passing conversation. That was when Linda noticed that Steven was shaking. "It started that day," Steven said, showing her his trembling hands, "and it won't stop." The image of Steven's hands stayed with Linda. A month later, while working on another story, Linda learned about work I was doing with a treatment technique called Eye Movement Desensitization and Reprocessing (EMDR).

EMDR is a psychological treatment designed for people who develop post-traumatic stress disorder (PTSD), an emotional response to severe trauma that changes the nervous system. EMDR uses special eye movements and other forms of brain stimulation to activate the whole brain, together with a stepwise process to remove the negative emotional charges on memories. With my colleagues Karen Lansing, Chris Hanks, and Lisa Rudy, I had just finished a study of six police officers involved in shootings who had developed PTSD. EMDR was very effective in alleviating the officers' symptoms, as well as normalizing brain function seen on SPECT scans.

CBS producer Angeline Chew called and asked if I would be interested in working on a story about EMDR, using Steven's story as an example. After talking to Steven, who was a willing participant, I recruited EMDR expert Sara Gilman to help. Sara is a seasoned trauma specialist and a close friend. We both interviewed Steven and felt he would be a good candidate for EMDR and that his story was worth telling through the eyes of EMDR and emotional healing. As in the case of most people who develop PTSD, the Santa Monica Farmers' Market disaster was not Steven's only trauma. He grew up in a severely abusive alcoholic home. One of his earliest memories is of his father burning down the family house. He also remembered that his father dangled him over a four-hundred-foot bridge. At the age of eleven his favorite uncle, a firefighter, died in a fire set by an arsonist, and Steven faced death as a tank commander during the Gulf War. Steven had many layers of trauma.

As part of his evaluation, we scanned Steven three times: before treatment, during his first EMDR session with Sara, and after eight hours of treatment. Initially, Steven's brain showed the classic PTSD pattern; his limbic or emotional brain was extremely hyperactive. Sara then went to work with him, cleaning out the traumas one by one using EMDR. His brain actually showed benefit during the first treatment and was markedly improved after only eight hours. His shaking subsided, and he felt significantly better. One of the most touching things Sara told me was that during the process Steven started to be able to forgive his father, and he even wondered what his father's brain would have looked like. He had held a deep and understandable resentment toward his father, but the work with brain science gave him a new perspective on himself and his father. When Sara and I helped him balance and change his brain, his life improved as well.

CATHY PLAYS ON TO HELP HER TEAM

One of my nieces (I have twenty-one nieces and nephews) is an amazing high school basketball player. Only five feet two inches tall, she played guard and helped lead her team to the state finals. Watching her play was one of the highlights of my life. One day my niece called me about a teammate, Cathy, who was about to be tossed off the basketball team. Cathy was a great player and an important part of the team, but she struggled with a terrible temper. She had problems with teammates and her coaches and frequently was thrown out of games because of negative interactions with referees. When Cathy came to see us, her scan showed two significant problems: low activity in her left temporal lobe (an area often associated with irritability and temper outburst) and increased activity in the anterior cingulate gyrus (often associated with arguing and trouble letting go of negative feelings and emotions). We put Cathy on some medications to balance her brain: an anticonvulsant to stabilize her temporal lobe and an antidepressant to calm her anterior cingulate gyrus. Within a month Cathy was more stable. Her temper was under control, and she became happier and more flexible. She was not thrown out of any more games and helped her team have an amazing year. As we helped balance and change Cathy's brain, she and her teammates were better off.

JIM IS BETTER THAN EVER

Jim, fifty-two, was the head of a large nonprofit support group. He was an able administrator and a loving husband and father, and he was successful in his other business endeavors. Over the two years before he came to see us, he noticed that his memory was not as good as it had been and that his energy level was waning. Jim heard me lecture at a science and technology conference in Washington, D.C., sponsored by the National Science Foundation. When he visited our clinic, it was clear that he was a successful, healthy male. Yet his brain was sleepy, which meant that it was underactive, especially in his prefrontal cortex and temporal lobes. These findings put him at risk for more serious problems later on. Based on his scan results, I put him on a handful of supplements and fish oil, changed his diet, and advised him to increase his exercise. We agreed that six months later we would get a follow-up scan to see how he was doing. The scan showed very nice overall improvement. Jim said he hadn't felt this good since he was in his twenties.

As you can see from these examples, it really is possible to change your brain and change your life. By enhancing brain function, you give yourself, your children, and your loved ones the best possible chance to be effective and happy in life.

THE MYTH OF THE PERFECT BRAIN

WE ALL NEED A LITTLE HELP

"The normal man is a fiction."

—Carl Jung

"The only normal people are the ones you don't know too well."

—Rodney Dangerfield

Jack is typical of many of the people who come to my clinics. Even though he was a competent, high-level computer executive, he struggled with his mood and temper. He was so ashamed of his shortcomings that he avoided getting help until his wife threatened to divorce him (a very common scenario in our clinics). When I first saw him, he said that he thought everyone else was normal except him, that everyone else was saner, better looking, and more confident, had more sex, and in general had a better time in life than he was having. As I listened, inwardly I smiled. A week with me, I thought, would completely dispel his notion that everyone else was normal. My next thought was a bit more sensitive. I remembered a time early in my psychiatric career when this odd thing kept happening to me. It seemed that anytime I got the idea that someone was really great, normal, healthy, and had it all together, within three weeks he would be in my office telling me about the pain, stress, traumas, sins, or disappointments in his own life. It happened so often that I started to believe that we all need a little help. Here are two brief examples.

One of the physicians at Fort Irwin, an army post in the middle of the

Mojave Desert where I spent two years as the chief of the community mental health center, had a barbecue at his house to welcome me when I first arrived at this isolated duty assignment. I met his wife and kids and had a wonderful time. I remember how much I admired him. Even though he was "very army" for a military doctor, he was smart and competent and seemed to truly care about the soldiers we were serving. Three weeks later his wife came to my office in tears and said how worried she was about his drinking. As it turned out, this physician had a serious drinking problem and was eventually sent to an inpatient program to get clean and sober.

One of my best friends through the years is a military chaplain. He is a kind, sensitive man with a big heart and a sharp wit. His soldiers love him, and he was rapidly promoted. I remember one particular day when I was thinking about how much I admired him (I need to stop having these thoughts), I got an urgent message that he had called. When I phoned him back, he was in a panic and had to see me right away. It was toward the end of the day, so I met him at the officers' club for dinner. I listened to him tell me about another side of himself well into the evening. During the day he had lost four hours of time and was afraid he was losing his mind. He did not know how he got to work or where his car was parked. And this was not the first time it had happened. It turned out that he had a multiple personality disorder from severe childhood abuse, which he didn't tell me about until he felt as though he was cracking up. I was saddened by his suffering and amazed at how functional he was given the multitude of traumas in his life.

A quick look at some of the statistics on mental illness will put to rest anyone's notion that the vast majority of people are without pain. According to the Epidemiological Catchment Study sponsored by the National Institute of Mental Health, 49 percent of the U.S. population at some point in their lives will suffer from a psychiatric (brain) illness, most commonly anxiety, depression, or substance abuse. Twenty-nine percent will have two psychiatric illnesses, and 17 percent will have three. Millions of people suffer, yet many think that others have it better. Most people have no idea how lucky they really are. It is normal to have struggles, and it is better to count your blessings than to feel messed up.

PRINCIPLE 9:
Very few people have perfect brains. We all need a little help.

When I first started my brain-imaging work, I was not very concerned with the concept of normal, because I had so many sick people to try to help. In our clinic's database, we have more than sixty murderers and hundreds of violent people. We have thousands of patients with ADD, anxiety, depression, brain trauma, substance abuse, and bipolar disorder. But building a database of normal people also became essential to my work. We needed normal people to do comparison studies on our patient group and to be able to understand and publish our results.

I knew that finding normal people would be a challenge. The people who I thought were normal often ended up in my office asking for help. Still, I had no idea how hard it would be to find truly normal brains. For our research project, we had fairly strict criteria for normal. This strictness was essential to our work and to being able to publish our studies. To be "normal" in our study, people had to meet five criteria:

- No psychiatric illness at any point in their lives (that eliminated 49 percent of the population),
- No significant head injuries,
- No substance abuse,
- No neurological problems, and
- No first-degree relative (mother, father, sibling, or child) with a psychiatric illness, including substance abuse problems.

Participants were thoroughly interviewed about the above issues and were given a structured psychiatric screening test, the Minnesota Multiphasic Personality Inventory (MMPI), which is a test of personality and a memory screening test.

I recruited people from within my own family (not the best place to start, except for my mother, who has a drop-dead-perfect brain), from my parents' country club, from churches and schools, by placing ads in the *Los Angeles Times,* and by placing flyers at local universities in student and teacher boxes. I even distributed flyers at my lectures (although there are not many normal mental health professionals). At the end of the second year of the study we had screened over fifteen hundred people and had scanned no more than sixty-five. Only about one in twenty-three people who thought they were normal actually met our criteria. Here are three examples of people who thought they were normal but actually were not.

Brad came to us as the fiancé of one of our employees. Everyone loved Brad. He was in school and worked and seemed like an all-around great guy. In the interview, however, it became clear that he struggled in school and that teachers thought he was not living up to his potential. He often procrastinated, was disorganized, had poor handwriting, and had experimented for three years with marijuana and cocaine. He never thought his substance abuse was a problem, so he didn't mention it until we pressed him on the subject.

Steve was a youth pastor who worked in a local church. He saw himself as kind, competent, and perfectly normal. His wife, on the other hand, saw him as temperamental, rigid, and moody. From his mother we found out that he had had a serious head injury as a child, where he fell backward from the top of a swing onto his head and sustained a brief loss of consciousness.

Gina seemed to meet all of our criteria and scored normally on our tests, except that she had some mild problems with the memory test. Her scan showed marked decreased activity in her prefrontal cortex. Puzzled, I interviewed her again. She had forgotten to tell me that she was being evaluated for chronic tiredness. She also cried very easily at emotional family events and even at commercials. She said, "It is definitely not normal to cry at KFC commercials showing a mother and son eating fried chicken together."

The research team was amazed that so many people who thought of themselves as not only normal but almost perfect were in reality troubled with mood or attentional problems or had histories of serious brain injury or forgotten substance abuse. As part of the screening process, we had spouses and parents fill out information on potential study subjects to make sure we always had another person's point of view.

Halfway through we changed the name of the study from the Amen Clinics Normal Study to the Amen Clinics Healthy Brain Study. Some may think that the name change was subtle, but we did not. We now believe that normal is a myth and healthy brains are actually rare. There are very few healthy brains among us. We all need a little help. This idea is actually comforting to me. It lessens judgment, because it is hard to say "I am better than you." It helps us see that brain health is fragile and must be taken seriously. And as a society, we need to make brain health a priority.

Along the same lines, we have found that many people who struggle do not know that they have problems. Did you know that 95 percent of people who have Alzheimer's disease are not diagnosed until they are in the moderate-to-severe stages of the illness? Clearly, it is much better to know that a problem is brewing early, so you can implement prevention and treatment strategies as soon as possible. Many people do not know that they have sustained brain injuries that have affected their lives. Many people also have no idea that they have mood or attentional problems; yet ask their spouses, and you will get an earful.

When I turned forty, I got a routine eye exam. To my surprise, I could not see past five feet out of my left eye. I was in serious need of glasses, yet I had had no idea. If we all need a little help, then early screening is an essential tool for keeping our brains healthy as we age.

PART II

THE AMEN CLINIC PROGRAM FOR MAKING A GOOD BRAIN GREAT

PROTECT YOUR BRAIN

The first step in making a good brain great is to work to protect it. Just as a parent shields a child from harm, you must take a proactive approach to keeping your brain safe from trouble. As simple as this idea is, most people never really think about brain security. We let those we love, including ourselves, snowboard without helmets, hit soccer balls with their heads, ride in unsafe cars, go off-roading in four-wheel vehicles, drink too much alcohol, smoke marijuana, consume drinks with excessive amounts of aspartame, sugar, or caffeine, become sleep deprived, and live with high levels of stress. Loving your brain means protecting it. I know many of you are thinking: *Oh no, more things I can't do—caffeine, alcohol, head injuries, paint fumes—why can't a person just have some fun?* Be careful, that is deprivation thinking. Just think, with a good brain, you can have better relationships, more love in your life, do more good for others, have more fun, be better at sports, have more sex, and be able to make and keep more money. It all depends on how you think about it. Without good functioning of your brain, trust me, you will not have more fun.

PROTECT YOUR BRAIN FROM PHYSICAL TRAUMA

After years of looking at the brain, I have concluded that protecting it is the first priority. I make sure my kids and loved ones drive safe vehicles, especially the youngest drivers. The young ones are at the greatest risk for harm, as their brains are not fully developed and they have more problems with impulsivity and poor judgment. As parents, we should read the safety ratings of vehicles, help our children get the safest cars, and strongly discourage them from riding motorcycles or mopeds.

Also, if possible—and they do not always listen—I would never let my children hit soccer balls with their heads or play tackle football or other sports that put them at risk for injuries. Some people have criticized me for being too protective. But it seems like a no-brainer (pun intended). One day my son-in-law, Jay, told me he was taking my daughter four-wheeling in California's desert. I protested. He said it was very safe and they are careful to wear helmets. I still protested. Sometimes knowing the truth still doesn't allow you to communicate it so others can see it as you do. A couple of months later they told me about an accident that brought shivers down my spine. Jay had been riding at forty miles per hour when the front tires of his four-wheel vehicle hit the top of a boulder buried in the sand. The accident launched Jay at forty miles per hour off the vehicle. How fast was his brain going while in midair? Forty miles per hour. He hit the sand helmeted-head first. His brain went from forty to zero in an instant. What do you think happened inside his skull? His brain bounced around multiple times. He was unconscious for a brief period of time. Given that he was then dating my daughter, I had already scanned him early in their relationship (sort of a rule in my family—take my daughter out for a while, get scanned to see if you can come back). Two months after the accident the scan showed a dent in his prefrontal cortex (Images 10.1 and 10.2). The four-wheeling was not exactly a smart idea. Both kids now get it. Protecting the brain from head injury is a critical part of being your best.

When it comes to sports, I often say, "Golf is good, tennis is terrific, table tennis is the world's best sport." Few head injuries occur with these sports, and both tennis and table tennis are highly aerobic. But when it comes to contact sports, despite a parent's pleading, some kids will still want to play. At this point, I believe children and teens should be screened for the apolipoprotein (apo) E4 gene. People who have this gene are 2.5 to 5 times more likely to develop Alzheimer's disease (AD). People who have this gene and also sustain a head injury have a tenfold risk of developing AD. If children or teens have the gene—and 25 percent of the population has it—there is no way in my mind that they should be allowed to play games where they might be injured. It is just too risky (Image 10.3).

Given the extraordinary increase in risk of AD when someone with the apoE4 gene has a head injury, it would be wise to know your apoE genotype before you decide whether to engage in high-risk activities. If you decide to

Jay's Brain

Image 10.1 Before Accident

Image 10.2 After Accident

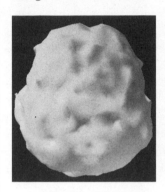

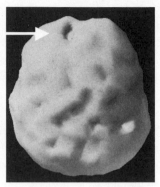

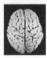

Healthy activity

Damage to right prefrontal area
(arrow)

Brain Trauma

Image 10.3 Underside View

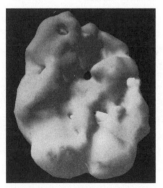

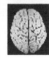

A sixteen-year-old boy in a bicycle
accident severely damaged his left
prefrontal cortex and temporal lobe

get an apoE genotype blood test, then it should be done under the strictest confidence so that insurance companies and others cannot obtain this information and potentially use it against you. It would be best to pay for the test on your own and keep it in your personal records, without allowing it to be included in your medical records.

Those who should consider getting an apoE genotype blood test include:

- Those who are considering playing contact sports where there is a high risk of injury to the head
- All professional athletes who engage in high-contact sports (boxing, football, soccer, hockey, etc.)
- Those with a brother, sister, father, or mother with AD
- People who sustained a head injury with loss of consciousness or who have had multiple head injuries

PROTECT YOUR BRAIN FROM EMOTIONAL TRAUMA AND STRESS

Emotional trauma, like physical trauma, can disrupt brain development and cause negative changes in the brain. We have studied many people who have been emotionally traumatized in fires, floods, earthquakes, and car accidents. We have studied people who have been robbed, raped, stabbed, shot, molested, and ritually tortured. We have seen policemen and firefighters who have been traumatized by losing friends during emergencies and having babies die in their arms. Emotional trauma changes brain function.

Our studies of emotional trauma indicate that the brain responds to trauma by firing up or flaming certain brain systems. Scans show that the deep limbic system, anterior cingulate gyrus, basal ganglia, and right temporal lobes all become hyperactive. It is as if all systems become hyperalert to be on guard for further trouble. When people have been traumatized, they have trouble sleeping, become moody, fearful, and anxious, and experience many physical "motor overflow" symptoms, such as headaches, muscle tension, or bowel problems. In addition, they are exposed to high levels of stress hormones, which have a direct negative effect on brain function. Chronic or lasting stress releases certain hormones that have been found to kill cells in the hippocampus, one of the major memory centers located in the temporal lobes. Stress from having too much to do, day in and day out, or from having unresolved emotional trauma clearly hurts brain function.

Protecting the brain from emotional trauma, and learning how to deal with chronic stress, are critical to brain health. In Chapter 18 we will discuss destressing the brain. For now, it is important to understand that stress and trauma hurt the brain, and that taking an active role in protecting the brain is critical to health.

For people who have been traumatized in the past I often refer them for Eye Movement Desensitization and Reprocessing (EMDR; see Chapter 8). This specific psychological treatment for trauma has been found to be effective not only in alleviating the symptoms of emotional trauma but also in re-balancing brain function. We performed a study of six police officers who were involved in shootings and subsequently developed post-traumatic stress disorder. PTSD is characterized by insomnia, nightmares, reliving the trauma, feeling emotionally numb, feeling that your life is shortened, and frequently intense anxiety. These officers were suffering both physical and emotional symptoms secondary to the trauma. We scanned each of the officers three times, before, during, and after treatment. All the officers showed dramatic improvement during the treatment process. In addition, the scans revealed that the treatment significantly helped brain function. You can learn more about EMDR at www.emdria.org.

Be watchful for too much stress and for traumatic events. Make sure to get the trauma treated and have a mechanism to lower the stress in your body.

PROTECT YOUR BRAIN FROM TOXIC EXPOSURE

Toxic exposure, like injury, emotional trauma, and stress, hurts the brain. Many substances have the potential to be brain toxic, and most people have no clue that they do. From many medications to drugs of abuse, from alcohol to caffeine (uh-oh, I may upset some folks here), from nicotine to environmental toxins, and from vaccines to pesticides, there are many things that can hurt your brain. Understanding the sources of brain poisons can help you avoid them.

Many medications are brain toxic. From a psychiatric standpoint, I was taught to use a class of antianxiety medications called benzodiazepines, such as Xanax, Ativan, and Valium, to treat patients with intense feelings of anxiety and panic. As soon as I started performing SPECT studies, I saw that these medications were often toxic to brain function. Scan after scan on these medications showed an overall diminished or dehydrated pattern of activity, just as with drugs of abuse, which we will discuss shortly. It didn't take long for me to stop using these medications and look for other ways to heal anxiety and panic. In much the same way, pain-killers often showed brain toxicity on scans: Vicodin, Darvon, Percodan, Oxycontin, and others caused overall decreased brain activity. No wonder they help pain—they make people feel numb all over. Of course, this doesn't mean that these medications are never indicated. Many people would rather die than live with chronic pain. It does mean, however, that we should look for other ways to work with chronic pain, rather than just giving pain-killers that also numb the brain. We should look toward acupuncture, hypnosis, biofeedback, herbs, and behavioral treatments to deal with pain. Whenever you take a medication, check to see the effect it has on the brain. Cognitive impairment is often spelled out in the side-effect profile given to patients by pharmacists.

Many patients who are on eight to ten different medications have come to see me complaining of memory problems. If I see trouble on their scans, my first goal is to decrease the number of medications they are taking. I have been amazed at how helpful that can be. One of my favorite patients came to me on eight different medications. Her frontal lobes were severely decreased in activity, and she had trouble forming her words. By better targeting her treatment, I was able to stop six of her medications and lower the doses of the two others. Her speech got better, her thought processes became clearer, and she had better energy than she had had in years. Her follow-up scan showed marked improvement.

Well-informed people understand clearly that drugs of abuse hurt the brain, but others debate it and argue. Drugs of abuse include alcohol, cocaine, methamphetamines, heroin, inhalants (the worst), marijuana, LSD, Ecstasy, and many others. When I first started to order scans, I was the director of a dual-diagnosis (mixed substance abuse and psychiatric disorder) treatment unit. I have seen well over a thousand scans of drug abusers (e.g., Image 10.4). The vast majority of them showed significant damage. More than 115 scientific studies have demonstrated the negative effects of drugs on the brain. The scans prove it. Through the years I have been grateful for my overall lack of substance and alcohol use. The scans had such powerful effects on my patients that I brought them home to show my children. I effectively induced anxiety disorders related to substance abuse in all of my children. I am happy that none of them has had a problem with drugs or alcohol, despite a significant family history of alcoholism on their mother's side. The power of the images led me to develop and be part of a series of posters and videos on substance abuse. *The Truth About Drinking,* produced

Drug Abuse Brain

Image 10.4 Top-Down View

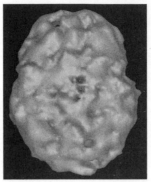

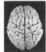

A twenty-two-year-old with alcohol
and cocaine abuse; overall scalloped,
toxic appearance to brain

by Arnold Shapiro and hosted by Leeza Gibbons, won an Emmy for best educational television program in 1998. Our poster, "Which Brain Do You Want," now hangs in over fifteen thousand schools. The images are very clear: alcohol and drugs damage the brain—stay away from them.

One of the most common brain toxins is alcohol. At the Amen Clinics we have seen many alcoholics, and they have some of the worst brains of all. Alcohol affects the brain by reducing nerve cell firing; it prevents oxygen from getting into the cells' energy centers; and it reduces the effectiveness of many different types of neurotransmitters, especially those involved in learning and remembering. Alcohol is a double-edged sword, depending upon the quantity of intake. Large amounts of it—four or more glasses of wine, or the equivalent in hard liquor on a daily basis—increase the risk of dementia. But small amounts—a glass of wine once a week or once a month, but not daily—may *reduce dementia by up to 70 percent*. The reduced risk seems to be related to the fact that alcohol and cholesterol compete with each other, and sometimes it is good for alcohol to win. That is, small amounts of alcohol compete with HDL, the good cholesterol, which actually removes the harmful types of cholesterol. When a person drinks a little alcohol, HDL is not allowed to bind to the cell membrane, so it is forced back into the bloodstream, where it lowers LDL and other harmful cholesterols. This reduces the person's risk of heart disease, atherosclerosis, and strokes, all of which are known causes for dementia. On the other hand, a recent study from Johns Hopkins reported that even small amounts of daily drinking lowered overall brain size. When it comes to the brain, size matters! My advice is that small amounts of alcohol after age twenty-five are okay, but don't push it. Why wait until you're twenty-five to drink? The brain is not fully developed until then, especially in the prefrontal judgment area. Why poison it before it has had a chance to fully develop?

Nicotine prematurely ages the brain. Nicotine, found in cigarettes, cigars, and chewing tobacco and in nicotine patches, tablets, and gum, causes blood vessels to constrict, lessening blood flow to vital organs. Smokers have more problems with impotence; it is bad to have low blood flow to sexual organs. Nicotine constricts blood flow to the skin, making smokers look prematurely older than they are. Nicotine also constricts blood flow to the brain, eventually causing overall lowered activity and depriving the brain of the nutrients it needs. If nicotine is so bad, then why do people smoke? In the short run nicotine, like alcohol and other drugs of abuse, makes many people feel better. It stimulates the release of several brain neurotransmitters, such as acetylcholine, which improves your reaction time and your ability to pay attention; dopamine, which acts in the pleasure center of the brain, reinforcing its use; glutamate, which is involved with learning and memory (although high glutamate levels cause programmed cell death and are involved in causing Alzheimer's disease); and endorphins, which are often called the body's natural pain-killer. No wonder people use nicotine and have trouble quitting. But if you want a healthy brain, do what you can to stay away from it.

Unfortunately, caffeine is not much better. Caffeine also constricts blood flow to the brain and many other organs. A little caffeine a day is probably not a problem, but more than a cup or two can certainly be trouble. Am I the only one worried about the proliferation of coffee companies? New coffee shops have seemed to spring up on every street corner, selling highly caffeinated drinks filled with sugar and fat. As a society, we are going from one or two cups a day to one or two cups three or four times a day. Why do so many people consume so much caffeine? Understanding the drug's actions can help us see why people use it so much and why we should significantly curb our use.

Adenosine, a chemical in the brain that causes drowsiness by slowing down nerve cell activity, is a key to understanding caffeine addiction. When we are tired, adenosine triggers the brain to slow down so we will go to sleep and naturally rejuvenate brain function. The purpose of sleep is to replenish certain chemicals in the brain to help with efficient nerve cell firing. Adenosine tells us when we need to sleep. Caffeine blocks the effects of adenosine by occupying the adenosine receptor sites and preventing the brain from seeing it. So even if you are tired and are in need of sleep to rejuvenate your brain chemistry, caffeine tricks the brain into thinking it is wide awake. Several sleep researchers suggest that we are a sleep-deprived nation and that caffeine addiction is a leading cause. Caffeine, a stimulant, causes the release of adrenaline from the adrenal glands, putting the body into a fight-or-flight mode, where the pupils dilate, the heart beats faster, blood vessels on the skin's surface constrict to slow blood flow from cuts and also to increase blood flow to muscles, blood pressure rises, blood flow to the stomach slows, the liver releases sugar into the bloodstream for extra energy, and muscles tighten up, ready for action. Caffeine puts us in a "ready state" for trouble.

Caffeine also increases dopamine levels in the same way that amphetamines do. Dopamine is a neurotransmitter that, in certain parts of the brain, activates the pleasure center. Obviously, caffeine's effect is much less than that of amphetamines, but the mechanism is similar. The dopamine/pleasure center connection may contribute to caffeine addiction. It is easy to see why your body likes caffeine in the short term, especially if you are sleep-deprived and need to stay active. Caffeine blocks adenosine receptors, so you feel alert. It raises adrenaline in your body, giving you a boost. And it raises dopamine production to make you feel good. The problem with caffeine is that it leads to a downhill spiral. Once the effects wear off, you feel fatigued and depressed. So you take more caffeine to get going again. As you might think, having your body in a constant state of readiness isn't very healthy, and you tend to feel jumpy and irritable. The most important long-term problem is the effect caffeine has on sleep. As we have seen, adenosine is important to sleep, especially to deep sleep. Significant caffeine consumption may prevent you from falling and staying asleep. Sleep deficits add up quickly, so the next day you feel worse and need caffeine to get out of bed. The cycle continues day after day. Ninety percent of Americans consume caffeine every day. Like other drugs of abuse, once you get in the cycle, you have to keep taking the drug. Even worse, if you try to stop taking caffeine, you get very tired and depressed and you get a terrible splitting headache. These negative effects force you back to caffeine even if you want to stop.

As little caffeine as possible is a good rule, if you want to respect and nurture your brain.

CAFFEINE CONTENT

According to the National Soft Drink Association, the caffeine content of soda (in milligrams, per 12-oz. can) is as follows:

Red Bull	80 (per 250 ml)
Jolt	71.2
Sugar-Free Mr. Pibb	58.8
Pepsi One	55.5
Mountain Dew	55.0 (no caffeine in Canada)
Diet Mountain Dew	55.0
Surge	51.0
Coca-Cola	45.6
Shasta Cola	44.4
Shasta Cherry Cola	44.4
Shasta Diet Cola	44.4
Mr. Pibb	40.8
Sunkist Orange	40
Dr Pepper	39.6
Pepsi Cola	37.2
Diet Pepsi	35.4
RC Cola	36.0
Canada Dry Cola	30.0
Barq's Root Beer	23
Canada Dry Diet Cola	1.2
7-Up	0
Diet Rite Cola	0
Sprite	0
Mug Root Beer	0
Diet Barq's Root Beer	0
Minute Maid Orange	0
A&W Root Beer	0

Coffee (6-oz. serving)	
Espresso	100
Brewed	80–135
Instant	65–100
Decaf, brewed	3–4

Decaf, instant	2–3
Tea, iced (12 oz.)	70
Tea, brewed, U.S.	40
Tea, instant	30
Herbal	0 (may vary)

Since many people have trouble judging portion sizes, here are the amounts of caffeine in Starbucks standard servings (in milligrams):

Coffee, grande (16 oz.)	550
Caffe Americano, short (8 oz.)	35
Coffee, tall (12 oz.)	375
Coffee, short (8 oz.)	250

Source: www.cspinet.org/nah/caffeine/caffeine_corner.htm

Another group of stimulants that are a source of concern is weight-loss supplements. Many of them contain high amounts of caffeine or caffeinelike substances. Now that ephedra is illegal, other herbal stimulants are gaining popularity, such as guarana, yerba maté, and cola nut, to name a few.

When it comes to toxic exposure, there are a number of controversial areas to consider. Some scientists report that mercury from any source is neurotoxic, such as the mercury found in certain fish, dental fillings, and the preservatives in vaccinations. In one study Dr. Hugh Fudenberg, one of the world's leading immunogeneticists, reported that people who have had five consecutive flu shots increased their risk of Alzheimer's disease tenfold compared to those who had one, two, or no shots. Dr. Fundenberg claimed it was due to the mercury and aluminum in flu shots. There is also great concern about the vaccinations we give to children: many of them contain the preservative thimerosal, which also contains mercury. Studies are conflicting, but why would we ever give children a known neurotoxin when other alternatives are available? In the 1950s kids routinely got five shots by the time they were two years old. Today's health guidelines call for more than twenty-two shots. Autism has risen more than twelvefold in the last decade. As some new studies have suggested, it is likely a genetic-toxin interaction. The genetic makeup of some children allows them to tolerate large doses of vaccinations containing mercury, while others do not. Clearly these are controversial areas. My advice is that less is more. If you don't need to do it, don't.

Artificial sweeteners are another area of concern. I have downed my share of diet drinks in my life, but when I read about the negative effects of artificial sweeteners, I get concerned. Many of my patients have felt better after stopping their intake of artificial sweeteners, and some have said their headaches went away, their joint pain improved, their memory improved, and surprisingly they lost weight. My sense is that it also depends on our own genetic makeup. Some people seem to have no problems with artificial sweeteners, while others have terrible reactions. Again, less is more.

Monosodium glutamate (MSG) is another problem for many. Personally, I get headaches and irritable when I eat something with MSG. But it is nothing like the reaction of one of my patients. This midwestern man came to see us with ADD and some anxiety and depressive symptoms. He told us he became violent when exposed to any MSG. We scanned him, and at his request we did an additional scan on MSG. The MSG scan showed a terrible left temporal lobe deficit, which is often associated with violence or rage reactions. I told him he had a choice: stay away from MSG, or take medication to protect his temporal lobes. To my surprise, he decided to take the medication just in case. When I asked why, he said that if he lost his temper one more time, his wife would leave him, and you never knew what had MSG in it. Whenever possible, hold the MSG.

Paint fumes and vapors from other solvents are brain toxins to avoid. As a group, indoor wall painters have some of the worst brains I have seen. I once evaluated a movie set director whose scan showed a toxic appearance. On questioning, it was clear he had been exposed to high levels of paint fumes on many of the sets he had worked on. Getting proper ventilation was one of the keys to helping him heal. In my conversation with him, he told me painters were the nuttiest people he ever worked with. He said they often got into fights for little to no reason and seemed unreliable. "Even the women act crazy," he said. No wonder, if they are exposed to chemicals that hurt the viability of brain tissue.

PROTECT YOUR BRAIN FROM SLEEP DEPRIVATION

Sleep deprivation from a number of causes also hurts the brain. People who get less than seven hours of sleep a night have lower activity in the temporal lobes, the part of the brain involved in learning and memory. Shift workers, those suffering from jet lag, teens who have their sleep schedules off-kilter from school schedules, and those suffering from sleep apnea are all at risk for poorer brain function. Those who are sleep-deprived score poorer on memory and math tests, have lower grades in school, and are at much greater risk for driving accidents. According to the National Highway Traffic Safety Administration, drowsiness and fatigue cause more than a hundred thousand traffic accidents each year, and young drivers are at the wheel in more than half the crashes. Sleep deprivation is also associated with depression and attention deficit disorders. Recently, sleep apnea (snoring loudly, holding breath when sleeping, and feeling tired during the day) has been linked to Alzheimer's disease.

Sleep is involved in rejuvenating the brain; without it, people can literally become psychotic. When I was chief of mental health at Fort Irwin, I saw a number of soldiers start to hear voices and become paranoid after being awake three days in a row. Fort Irwin is home to the national training center that teaches soldiers desert warfare. Troops spent days at a time in war games without much sleep. Mental health casualties were always high during those periods of time.

New research suggests that people who put on a few extra pounds may be able to blame lack of sleep for the added weight. Eve Van Cauter, a professor of medicine at the University of Chicago, coauthored a study reporting that people who are sleep-deprived eat more simple carbohydrates than people with good sleep. Sleep regulates two hormones, leptin and ghrelin, that are involved in appetite. People tend to replace reduced sleep with added calories. Van Cauter and colleagues wrote in the *Annals of Internal Medicine* that they studied twelve healthy men in their early twenties. They measured circulating levels of leptin and ghrelin before the study, after two nights of only four hours of sleep, and after two nights of ten hours of sleep. After four hours of sleep, the ratio of ghrelin jumped 71 percent, compared to a night when the men slept nine hours. The sleep-deprived men chose candy, cookies, and cake over fruit, vegetables, or dairy products.

A second study found that the less people sleep, the more they weigh, using a measure called body mass index, which scales weight to height. It also found lower leptin levels and higher ghrelin levels in people who sleep less. Dr. Emmanuel Mignot of Stanford University and colleagues examined a thousand people in the Wisconsin Sleep Cohort Study, measuring the participants' sleep habits, their sleep on the night before the exam, and their leptin and ghrelin levels. They found that people who consistently slept five hours or less per night had on average 14.9 more ghrelin and 15.5 percent lower leptin levels than those who slept eight hours a night. Both of these studies demonstrate an important relationship between sleep, appetite, and metabolic hormones.

Work to sleep at least seven or eight hours each night. Practice good sleep habits, such as avoiding much caffeine and nicotine; stay away from alcohol as a sleep aid, as it will wear off and cause you to wake up in the middle of the night; avoid exercise before bed; and learn relaxation techniques to calm your mind.

Protect your brain!

EAT RIGHT TO THINK RIGHT

FOOD AS BRAIN MEDICINE

I am what I ate . . . and I'm frightened.

—Bill Cosby

You are what you eat. Literally. All the cells in your body, including your brain cells, make themselves new every five months. Some, like your skin cells, make themselves new every month. Proper nutrition is critical to maintaining a healthy brain and body. Food is as powerful as any medicine that science can design. Intuitively, we know food has a powerful impact on how we feel. Eat right, and you feel better. Eat wrong, have three doughnuts to start your day, and you could end up feeling lethargic and stupid thirty to sixty minutes later. If you desire to have a great brain, you must give it consistent nutrition. This is one of the easiest, most effective strategies to get results quickly. This chapter will be your road map to eating for brain health.

The way we Americans feed ourselves and our children is scandalous. Just take breakfast, for example. Think of what we feed our children and ourselves: sugary cereals, muffins, doughnuts, frozen pancakes and waffles with liquid sugar (maple syrup), and cinnamon rolls. All these things are laden with calories, refined carbohydrates, and damaged fats that cause blood sugar spikes and drops that make us feel hungry and erratic throughout the day.

We are also exporting our poor eating habits to other countries. My wonderful friend in China, Tang Yiyuan, a scientist at the Chinese National Academy of Sciences, says the most popular restaurants in Beijing are American fast-food restaurants. As the Chinese diet is starting to resemble the American diet, he says, they are seeing an increased incidence of illnesses, such as diabetes and heart disease. Given what we know about nutrition, health, and illness, it is neglectful or even self-abusive to eat the standard American diet, which has too many refined carbohydrates, too much bad fat, and way too many calories (many of which are empty and toxic).

As a society, Americans are constantly bombarded with advertisements that promote sales and encourage illness:

> Do you want to "go large" with your order? It's only thirty-nine cents!
> Do you want fries with your meal?
> Do you want an appetizer?
> Do you want bread first [which makes you hungrier so you eat more]?
> Do you want dessert? It comes with the meal!
> Do you want another drink? A bigger drink? It is a better deal!
> You get toys with the children's meals!
> Happy hour—you can drink more for less!
> If you're good I'll take you for French fries or get you dessert. [Poor nutrition as a reward for good behavior sets us up later in life to reward ourselves with food that is not good for us.]
> Free refills, bottomless fries, all-you-can-eat buffets [I have to keep eating to get my money's worth].

When the fast-food restaurant says "Do you want to go large?" say no. Why pay extra money to be fat and have less brain function?

One group of people who need to have the best diets are teenagers and young adults, as their brains are still developing. Unfortunately, they are famous for having the worst diets. Many teens and young adults have little education in nutrition and give in to their desires for "bottomless fries" or "supersized meals" without thinking about the consequences. Because of their underdeveloped prefrontal lobes, teens succumb to their impulses and eat whatever they want, whatever tastes good, whatever is on the table. Yet teenage obesity and adult-onset diabetes in teens are reaching epidemic proportions. The teenage and young adult brain is going through vast changes, and giving it proper nutrition helps to build better adults. Parents and schools need to take an active role in teaching kids how to eat, not just abdicate our role because we think our teenagers won't listen to us. My experience with three teenagers and hordes of their friends is that if you educate them, give them tasty, healthful options, and gently nudge them in the right direction, they make better choices.

An important concept to remember here is that exposure equals preference. With the food you provide for them at home, you are teaching your kids what to like and therefore what to choose to eat. Expose your kids to a wide variety of healthy choices so that they will learn to like the right food and make good choices when they are away from you.

SEVEN SIMPLE BRAIN-PROMOTING NUTRITIONAL TIPS

Here is the seven-step plan to get your diet under control and to use food as brain medicine.

1. INCREASE WATER INTAKE

Given that your brain is about 80 percent water, the first rule of brain nutrition is to hydrate your brain with adequate water. Even slight dehydration can raise stress hormones, which can damage your brain over time. Drink at least 84 ounces of water a day. It is best to have your liquids unpolluted with artificial sweeteners, sugar, caffeine, or alcohol. Actually, caffeine is a diuretic and causes dehydration, which works against your brain's need for water. But you do not necessarily need to have all the water plain. As you'll see in health spas, you can add pieces of fruit, such as lemons, limes, or oranges, to water to get a hint of flavor. You can also use herbal, noncaffeinated teabags, such as raspberry- or strawberry-flavored, and make unsweetened iced tea. Green tea is also good for brain function, as it contains chemicals that enhance mental relaxation and alertness.

2. CALORIE RESTRICTION

Substantial research in animals and now in humans indicates that a calorie-restricted diet is helpful for brain and life longevity. Eating less helps you live longer. It controls weight; it decreases risk for heart disease, cancer, and stroke from obesity (a major risk factor for all of these illnesses); and it triggers certain mechanisms in the body to increase the production of nerve growth factors, which are helpful to the brain. Researchers use the acronym *CRON* for "calorie restriction with optimal nutrition," so the other part of the story is to make these calories count.

Personally, I hate this principle. I love to eat. My grandfather, whose name I carry, was a candy maker. My earliest, happiest childhood memories are of being five years old standing on a step stool at the stove in my grandfather's home making fudge, English toffee, and pralines. I can still smell the candy cooking. It is comfort food for me, but it also makes my mind foggy and slow. Additionally I am handicapped by a mother who is an amazing Lebanese cook. I love her cooking, such as cabbage or grape leaves rolled and stuffed with lamb, rice, and allspice, cooked in a tomato-based broth; freshly baked pizza with onions, mushrooms, and sausage; or Syrian bread warm out of the oven, dripping in butter. The list goes on and on. I love her cooking, but I hate the idea of being fat; this is a serious emotional conflict. My father says he has to get mad at my mom when she cooks such wonderful meals, which she loves to do whenever one or more of her twenty-one grandchildren come to visit. I have heard my father say to her, "It is like having a beautiful naked woman sitting on the counter and saying 'Don't touch.' It just isn't going to happen."

Even though I hate the idea of "eat less, live longer," it is what research tells us to do, and it makes good sense. So grudgingly I strive to eat fewer than eighteen hundred calories a day, and I recommend you do the same. Figure out how many calories you need to stay at your weight or even lose weight if that is your desire, and then go a little bit below it. I watch what I eat, know the calorie content of the food I put in my mouth, and even weigh portions when I am not sure. One of my big fears in life was that I would become short, fat, and bald. I am only five foot six, and people tend to get shorter with age after forty. I started to go bald in my twenties, like my grandpa the candy maker. So the only thing I have control over is my weight. I have a brother, whom I adore, who is a hundred pounds overweight. I worry more about his health than he does, but I know that if I ate whatever I wanted, I would be wearing parachutes for shorts and suffer from knee and back pain as he does.

3. FISH, FISH OIL, GOOD FATS, AND BAD FATS

Recently, while on vacation in Alaska, I saw a bumper sticker that read, "Fish Control My Brain." I smiled when I realized that the saying had an element of truth to it, beyond the obsession with fishing. Fish as brain food? In fact, DHA, one form of the omega-3 fatty acids found in fish, makes up a large portion of the gray matter of the brain. The fat in your brain forms cell membranes and plays a vital role in how our cells function. Neurons are also rich in omega-3 fatty acids. DHA is also found in high quantities in the retina, the light-sensitive part of the eye. Research in the last few years has revealed that a diet rich in omega-3 fatty acids may help promote a healthy emotional balance and positive mood in later years, possibly because DHA is a main component of the brain's synapses. A Danish team of researchers compared the diets of 5,386 healthy older individuals and found that the more fish in a person's diet, the longer the person was able to maintain their memory. Dr. J. A. Conquer and his colleagues from the University of Guelph in Ontario studied the blood fatty acid content in the early and later stages of dementia and noted low levels in their subjects when compared to healthy people.

Since fish have a high content of omega-3 fatty acids, they can aid good brain health. In a well-designed study from Holland, researchers found that diets high in saturated fat and cholesterol increased dementia and stroke risk, while fish consumption decreased the chances of getting those illnesses. The researchers evaluated the food intake of 5,386 normal aging persons and followed them for 2.1 years. Those with a high intake of total fat, saturated fat, or cholesterol were, respectively, 2.4, 1.9, and 1.7 times more likely than those with a lower intake to develop dementia. Eating fish reduced dementia risk, especially that due to Alzheimer's disease. In a study published in the *British Medical Journal*, French researchers reported that older people who eat fish at least once a week have a significantly lower risk of developing brain problems. "There is an inverse relationship between the frequency of fish consumption and the incidence of dementia," according to the lead author, Dr. Pascale Barberger-Gateau. Older people who ate fish at least once a week had about a 33 percent decrease in dementia risk over seven years. Dr. Barberger-Gateau and colleagues evaluated fish, seafood, and meat consumption among 1,674 normal aging individuals over sixty-seven years old living in southwestern France. Over the seven years of follow-up, they found that increased fish and seafood consumption significantly reduced the chance of developing dementia. One concern about fish is the level of toxins, such as mercury, found in some species. Once or twice a week is a good policy. High-quality, purified fish oil is another option (see Chapter 20).

Five Reasons to Buy Wild Salmon

Many people know that wild salmon is better than farmed salmon. Here are five reasons why, as listed by the Sierra Club.

1. Farmed salmon pollute. They are raised in farms of floating net-pens. The immense accumulation of waste products can spoil the local environment and spread disease. In addition to natural wastes, farmed salmon are given antibiotics as well as other drugs that may harm humans and local ecosystems.

2. Farmed salmon escape. Storms, sea lions, and net breaks cause large releases of farmed salmon into the environment. A significant portion of salmon farmed in the Pacific are, in fact, Atlantic salmon. Escaped fish may ultimately compete with and displace native stocks.

3. Farmed salmon are expensive. Farmed salmon represent a net loss of protein, requiring three to five pounds of fish meal to yield a pound of salmon. Think about the energy expended to catch, process, and transport the fish meal, and "less expensive" salmon seem very expensive.

4. Eating wild salmon is better for you. Like livestock, farmed salmon are given the same antibiotics that are used to treat humans, a practice condemned by the World Health Organization for contributing to worldwide antibiotic resistance. Wild salmon are not only drug- and antibiotic-free, they also have higher levels of beneficial omega-3 fatty acids and lower levels of harmful saturated fats. According to the U.S. Department of Agriculture, farmed Atlantic salmon contain 70 percent more fat than wild Atlantic salmon and 200 percent more fat than wild Pacific pink and chum salmon. But perhaps most important, farm-raised salmon have been found to contain significantly higher concentrations of PCBs, dioxin, and other cancer-causing contaminants than salmon caught in the wild.

5. Wild salmon are tastier. They have better texture than farm-raised fish, which tend to be mushy and insipid. Without added dyes, farmed fish also lack the trademark color of natural salmon.

To get the very best salmon, buy it fresh and in season. The best choices include trawl-caught and Copper River salmon from Alaska. Most canned salmon is wild, but look on the label. Keep in mind that while many wild salmon runs are threatened, endangered, or even extinct, many are also still healthy. As a general rule, wild stocks in Alaska are faring far better than those of California and the Pacific Northwest. As for Atlantic salmon, there are virtually no harvestable wild runs left in the United States.

Given the recent data on the healthful effects of eating fish and omega-3 fatty acids, it is reasonable to increase the amount of fish in your diet or take a daily fish oil, omega-3 fatty acid supplement. If you do take a fish oil supplement, you need to ensure that it has been tested for contaminants and heavy metals and protected from oxidation during the processing so that it doesn't get rancid. (For more on fish oil and omega-3 fatty acid supplements, see Chapter 20.)

Many myths and misconceptions surround dietary fat, which has resulted in a widespread fat phobia, although this has lessened with the popularity of low-carb diets. It is important to remember that not all fat is bad, and that some is essential. The solid weight of your brain is 60 percent fat. The hundred billion nerve cells in the cerebral cortex require essential fatty acids to function. Myelin, the white fatty covering on the axons of nerve cells that speed the conduction of electrical impulses, is extremely important for the well-being of the nervous system. Amyotrophic lateral sclerosis (ALS), commonly known as Lou Gehrig's disease, and multiple sclerosis (MS) are called demyelinating diseases, because a loss of myelin is the essential feature. Certainly high-circulating fat can kill you with heart disease and strokes, but too-low fat levels can also cause problems such as depression and anger, sometimes even suicide and homicide.

There are two main categories of fat—good fat (the unsaturated kind) and bad fat (the saturated kind). Saturated fats are molecules whose binding sites are literally saturated or filled with hydrogen molecules. They are stiff and contribute to hardening of the arteries and cholesterol plaques. Saturated fats are found in red meat, eggs, and dairy foods (like butter and milk). They do not spoil as easily as their healthier counterparts, the unsaturated fats. There are also fats that have been chemically altered by adding hydrogen so that they act like saturated fats; these are called partially hydrogenated oils. The food industry uses them because they do not oxidize and get rancid, but you should stay away from them, as they are more damaging than saturated fats and belong in a special category all their own, known to critics as "Frankenfats."

The binding sites of unsaturated fats (mono- or polyunsaturated) are not fully saturated by hydrogen and are more flexible, which is why unsaturated fats melt at a lower temperature than saturated fats. They rot more easily when exposed to air, they metabolize more easily, and they lower blood cholesterol levels. Monounsaturated fats lower LDL cholesterol, the type of cholesterol that makes a major contribution to hardening the arteries. Monounsaturated fats also raise HDL cholesterol, which protect against cardiovascular disease. While polyunsaturated fats also provide the beneficial effect of lowering LDL cholesterol, they also lower HDL cholesterol, which is not good. The monounsaturated fats are therefore preferred over the polyunsaturated fats. Monounsaturated fats are found in avocados, nuts (such as almonds, cashews, and pistachios), canola oil, olive oil, and peanut oil. Polyunsaturated fats are found in safflower oil, corn oil, and some fish.

The polyunsaturated fats found in salmon and mackerel, and the monounsaturated fats found in canola oil and soybean oil, are high in the essential fatty acids (EFA) called omega-3 fatty acids. EFAs cannot be made by the human body and therefore must be obtained from diet (hence the name *essential* fatty acids). Omega-3 fatty acids are considered good fat because they are important components of our cells and the cell membranes that are essential for life and health.

It is hard to get enough omega-3 fatty acids into our diet. The fast and processed foods that are now part of our everyday diets are often deficient in them. Even if your diet includes several meals of fish per week, you still may not be ingesting sufficient amounts of omega-3. This is because much of the fish we consume is now farm raised or does not contain significant amounts of omega-3. When you are ordering fish in a restaurant or buying it at the store, ask if it was caught in the wild or farm raised. Ideally, adults should consume at least 900 mg of long-chain omega-3 (DHA + EPA) per day, either from food sources or dietary supplementation. (For information on DHA and EPA, see page 198.) Omega-3 fatty acids are found in deep, coldwater fish, such as salmon, mackerel, and sardines. Omega-6 fatty acids are also important but are usually found in adequate amounts in corn, safflower, sunflower, and soybean oils.

Flaxseed oil is not as good a source of omega-3, because your body has to convert its omega-3 fatty acid (alpha-linolenic acid, or ALA) to DHA. This conversion can be inefficient, and some people of specific ethnic backgrounds or who suffer from diabetes may not be able to convert from ALA to DHA at all. Fish, however, do the work for us by converting omega-3 to DHA and EPA. You can therefore eat less fish than flaxseed oil and still get what your body needs.

Heart disease was the first area investigated with regard to the health impact of omega-3 fatty acids. In the early 1970s researchers noticed that the Inuit people of Greenland had a high-fat, high-cholesterol diet yet were able to maintain healthy hearts. Subsequent investigations concluded that this was due to the high level of omega-3 fatty acids in their native diet of fish and marine animals. Since then several other studies, including two large American studies in 1997 and 1998, have revealed the same thing: that cardiovascular health is enhanced in weekly fish eaters when compared to those who ate fish only infrequently. **Don't forget: Whatever is good for your heart is also good for your brain!**

GOOD FATS VERSUS BAD FATS

Good Fats (most are high in omega-3)	Bad Fats (most are high in omega-6)
Anchovies	Bacon
Avocados	Butter
Brazil nuts	Cheese (regular fat)
Canola oil	Cream sauces
Cashews	Doughnuts
Flaxseed oil	Fried foods, such as
Green leafy vegetables	potatoes/onion rings
Herring	Ice cream
Lean meats	Lamb chops
Low-fat cheeses	Low-carbohydrate bars
Olive oil	Margarine
Peanut oil	Potato chips (fried)
Pistachio nuts	Processed foods
Salmon	Steak
Sardines	Whole milk
Soybean oil	
Trout	
Tuna	
Walnuts	
Whitefish	

4. LOTS OF DIETARY ANTIOXIDANTS

A number of studies have shown that dietary intake of antioxidants from fruits and vegetables significantly reduces the risk of developing cognitive impairment. The research was done because it was theorized that free radical formation plays a major role in the deterioration of the brain with age. When a cell converts oxygen into energy, tiny molecules called free radicals are made. When produced in normal amounts, free radicals work to rid the body of harmful toxins, thereby keeping it healthy. When produced in toxic amounts, free radicals damage the body's cellular machinery, resulting in cell death and tissue damage. This process is called oxidative stress. Vitamins E and C and beta-carotene inhibit the production of free radicals. Working independently on two continents, researchers in Rotterdam and in Chicago found evidence to support these hypotheses.

Good sources of vitamin C are tomatoes, fruits (especially citrus and kiwi), melon, raw cabbage, green leafy vegetables, peppers, sprouts, broccoli, and cabbage. Important sources of vitamin E are grains, nuts, milk, egg yolk, wheat germ, vegetable oils, and green leafy vegetables.

Blueberries (also called brain berries) are an especially good source of antioxidants. A series of studies feeding blueberries to rats have examined the berries' effects on learning new motor skills as well as protection against stroke. Rats that were fed blueberries better learned new motor skills as they aged compared to their study counterparts. Rats fed a blueberry-enriched diet that were then given a stroke (in the name of science) lost only 17 percent of the neurons in their hippocampus, compared to 42 percent neuron loss in rats not eating blueberries.

Strawberries and spinach have also shown significant protective effects in rat models, although not as strongly as blueberries. In addition, the rats receiving these antioxidant-enriched diets all showed increased levels of vitamin E in their brains. "The exciting finding from this study is the potential reversal of some age-related impairment in both memory and motor coordination, especially with blueberry supplements," said Molly Wagster, Ph.D., a health science administrator with the National Institute of Aging.

THE BEST ANTIOXIDANT FRUITS AND VEGETABLES (ACCORDING TO THE U.S. DEPARTMENT OF AGRICULTURE)

Blueberries
Blackberries
Cranberries
Strawberries
Spinach
Raspberries

Brussels sprouts
Plums
Broccoli
Beets
Avocados
Oranges
Red grapes
Red bell peppers
Cherries
Kiwis

Eat from the rainbow (many colors) of fruits and vegetables to ensure that you are getting a wide variety of antioxidants to nourish and protect your brain.

5. A BALANCE OF PROTEIN, GOOD FATS, AND CARBOHYDRATES

Given the weight issues in my family, I have read many of the diet books that are popular in America. Some I like a lot, while others make me a little crazy. Eating protein and fat only and avoiding most grains, fruits, and vegetables may be a quick way to lose weight, but it is not a healthy long-term way to eat for your body or your brain. The best thing about the Atkins Diet and its many clones is that it gets rid of most simple sugars. Diets high in refined sugars, such as the low-fat diets of the past, encourage diabetes, tiredness, and cognitive impairment. Yet to imply that bacon is a health food and that oranges and carrots are as bad as cake seems silly. The more balanced diets, such as *The Zone* by Barry Sears, *Sugar Busters!* by H. Leighton Steward and a group of Louisiana-based physicians, *The South Beach Diet* by cardiologist Arthur Agatston, and *Powerful Foods for Powerful Minds and Bodies* by René Thomas make sense from a body and brain perspective. The main principle to take away from these programs is that balance is essential, especially balancing proteins, good fats, and good carbohydrates. Having protein at each meal helps to balance blood sugar levels; and adding lean meat, eggs, cheese, soy, or nuts to a snack or meal limits the fast absorption of carbohydrates and prevents the brain fog that goes with eating simple carbohydrates, such as doughnuts. In fact, psychologist Keith Connors of Duke University found that adding protein to the breakfast of ADD children improved the effectiveness of their medication. Limiting most carbohydrates to those with a low glycemic index (such as nuts, apples, pears, and beans), which measures how quickly blood sugar and insulin rise in response to a food, allows one to get the energy and nutrients of carbohydrates, and the brain to use the carbohydrates exclusively for fuel, without bingeing or overeating them. And consuming healthy fats, such as those with higher levels of omega-3 fatty acids, makes for balanced meals and balanced minds. At each meal or snack, try to get a balance of protein, high-fiber carbohydrates, and fat.

In 2000 I did a study with five ADD college students, including my own son, using the *Zone* diet plus high-dose purified fish oil. Each teen stayed on this regimen for five months. We tracked their school performance and did before-and-after brain SPECT scans. All the students performed better in school, and all lost weight. In fact, one girl complained that she lost so much weight that her breasts were significantly smaller. (Breast tissue is primarily fat tissue.) Their scans showed positive changes as well, calming overactive areas involved in mood control and enhancing the concentration centers of the brain. Diet and fish oil help to balance brain function. The nice thing about this approach is that there are no side effects; unlike the medications used to help balance brain function, which sometimes are clearly needed, diet and fish oil have no downside!

Critics of the higher-protein diets say that the brain exclusively uses carbohydrates for energy, which is true. But they forget that protein is an essential component of nerve cells, axons, and dendrites—the machinery of the brain. Low-protein diets leave the brain without critical resources. Neuroscientist Marian Diamond had an experience in Kenya that stimulated important research. She found that pregnant women would not eat protein because it meant they would have to deliver a larger baby. It was much easier, in their view, to reduce their protein intake to ensure a smaller baby and an easier delivery. Dr. Diamond then wondered about the effect of reduced protein intake on a developing infant's brain. That became the subject of a series of experiments in her laboratory as soon as she returned home to Berkeley. One of her graduate students, Arianna Carughi, fed half the pregnant rats a normal high-protein diet and the other half a low-protein diet. The body weight of the babies whose mothers had been fed the reduced-protein diet was found to be 50 percent less than that of the babies whose mothers had been given a normal protein diet. And the brains? The dendrites in the reduced-protein baby rats did not develop fully. When they placed the protein-deprived babies in an enriched learning environment, their dendrites did not increase significantly, as they did in the normal-protein babies living in an enriched environment. It is clear that a protein-rich diet is vital for growing healthy nerve cells that can respond positively to enriched living conditions. Protein is essential to brain growth.

6. PICK YOUR TOP TWENTY-FOUR HEALTHY FOODS, AND PUT THEM IN YOUR DIET EVERY WEEK

To stick with a "brain healthy" calorie-restricted nutritional plan, you must have great choices. I am fond of the book *Super Foods Rx* by Steven Pratt and Kathy Matthews, which lists fourteen top food groups that are healthy and reasonable in calories. I have added several more choices (indicated by a double asterisk) that are especially good for the brain. Choose from among these twenty-four foods each week. They are healthy, low in calories, powerful in antioxidants, lean in protein, and rich in high-fiber carbohydrates and good fat.

The American Cancer Society recommends five to nine servings of fruits and vegetables a day. Mixing colors (eating from the rainbow) is a good way to think about consuming healthy fruits and vegetables. Strive to eat red things (strawberries, raspberries, cherries, red peppers, and tomatoes), yellow things (squash, yellow peppers, small portions of bananas and peaches), blue things (blueberries), purple things (plums), orange things (oranges, tangerines, and yams), green things (peas, spinach, and broccoli), and so on.

Lean Protein
1. Fish—salmon (especially Alaskan salmon caught in the wild; farmed fish are not as rich in omega-3 fatty acids), tuna, mackerel, herring (also listed under Fats)
2. Poultry—chicken (skinless) and turkey (skinless)
3. Meat—lean beef and pork
4. Eggs (enriched DHA eggs are best)
5. Tofu and soy products (whenever possible, choose organically raised)
6. Dairy products—low-fat cheeses and cottage cheese, low-fat sugar-free yogurt, and low-fat or skim milk
7. Beans, especially garbanzo beans and lentils (also listed under Complex Carbohydrates)

8. Nuts and seeds, especially walnuts (also listed under Fats). Great recipe: soak walnuts in water and sea salt overnight, drain and sprinkle with cinnamon (a natural blood sugar balancer), and low-roast four hours at 250° F—it makes them easier to digest.

Complex Carbohydrates

9. Berries—especially blueberries (brain berries), raspberries, strawberries, and blackberries
10. Oranges, lemons, limes, grapefruit
11. Cherries
12. Peaches, plums
13. Broccoli, cauliflower, Brussels sprouts
14. Oats, whole wheat, wheat germ. Oatmeal should be the long-cooking kind, as instant has a higher glycemic index—the manufacturer breaks down the fiber to speed the cooking time and basically makes it a refined carbohydrate. The same goes for bread—look for at least three grams of fiber. Remember that unbleached wheat flour is white flour—the label must say whole wheat.
15. Red or yellow peppers (much higher in vitamin C than green peppers)
16. Pumpkin squash
17. Spinach—works wonderfully as a salad, or a cooked vegetable; adds fiber and nutrients
18. Tomatoes
19. Yams
** Beans (also listed under Lean Protein)

Fats

20. Avocados
21. Extra-virgin cold-pressed olive oil
22. Olives
** Salmon (also listed under Lean Protein)
** Nuts and nut butter, especially walnuts, macadamia nuts, Brazil nuts, pecans and almonds (also listed under Lean Protein)

Liquids

23. Water
24. Green or black tea

7. PLAN SNACKS

I love to snack; I just like to munch on things to get through the day. When snacking, as I've said, it is helpful to balance carbohydrates, proteins, and fats. Since I travel frequently, I have learned to take my snacks with me, so I am not tempted to pick up candy bars along the way. One of my favorite low-calorie snacks is dried fruits and vegetables. I don't mean the kind of dried fruits and vegetables stocked in typical supermarkets, which are filled with preservatives. I mean the kind that just have the dried fruit and veggies. A company called Just Tomatoes, in Walnut, California (www.justtomatoes.com), makes great products. They make dried peaches (my favorite), strawberries (second favorite), mangoes, apples, cherries (fabulous), blackberries, blueberries (oh, so good), persimmons, and raspberries without anything added. They also make a product called Just Veggies that is a wonderfully sweet and crunchy snack of carrots, corn, peas, bell peppers, and tomatoes. It tastes like an unusual but wonderful popcorn and is as guiltless a snack as you will ever find. I keep some in my desk drawer and briefcase—perfect for those afternoon hunger attacks. When you have dried fruit or veggies—all carbohydrates—add some low-fat string cheese or a few nuts to balance it out with protein and a little fat.

- Deviled eggs with hummus: slice the eggs, discard the yolks, and fill with 1 tablespoon hummus; add paprika to taste.
- Low-fat cottage cheese with fruit and a couple of almonds or macadamia nuts
- Low-fat yogurt and nuts
- Ham and apple roll-up with a macadamia nut or three almonds
- 1 ounce of string cheese and a half cup of grapes

From the Barry Sears website www.drsears.com: you can create an infinite number of healthy brain snacks by mixing one item from each group.

PROTEINS

- ¼ cup low-fat cottage cheese
- 1 oz. part-skim or "lite" mozzarella
- 2½ oz. part-skim or "lite" ricotta cheese
- 1 oz. sliced meat (turkey, ham, etc.)
- 1 oz. tuna packed in water
- 1 oz. low-fat, part-skim, or "soft" cheese

CARBOHYDRATES

- ½ apple
- 3 apricots
- 1 kiwi
- 1 tangerine
- ⅓ cup "lite" fruit cocktail
- ½ pear
- 1 cup strawberries
- ¾ cup blackberries
- ½ orange
- ½ cup grapes
- 8 cherries
- ½ nectarine
- 1 peach
- 1 plum
- ½ cup crushed pineapple
- 1 cup raspberries
- ½ cup blueberries
- ½ grapefruit
- 1–2 Akmak or other whole-grain fat-free crackers

FATS

- 3 olives (green or black)
- 1 macadamia nut
- 1 tbsp. guacamole
- 3 almonds
- 6 peanuts
- 2 pecan halves
- 1 tbsp. almond butter

BRAIN-HEALTHY RECIPES

Here are some brain-healthy recipes I use frequently in my own life. My favorite is Dorie's Truly Amazing Lamb, Beans, and Rice. It was one of my favorite foods growing up. Originally it contained three times its current calorie count. My mother and I worked on the recipe to decrease the calories but keep the flavor. When I cooked it recently for a group of family and friends, every diner's plate was scraped clean. You can keep taste but get rid of calories—it just takes a little thought. Consistency is what counts with nutrition. Here are some suggestions.

BREAKFAST RECIPES

Berry Decadence (my favorite)

8 oz. frozen mixed berries (blueberries, raspberries, and blackberries)
6 oz. of nonfat sugar-free plain yogurt
¼ cup All-Bran cereal
1 tbsp. chopped walnuts (for crunch and omega-3 fatty acids)
1 tbsp. whey protein

Heat the frozen berries, then stir in the yogurt, cereal, walnuts, and protein. Eat warm. It tastes like pie filling but is very healthy, with three of our favorite foods.

Serves one
Calories—230

Sara's Low-Fat Southwestern Chicken Omelet

6 egg whites or Egg Beaters
½ chopped tomato, handful of mushrooms, onions to taste, 1 cup red
*   peppers*
3 oz. lean turkey or chicken
1 oz. mozzarella cheese
extra-virgin olive oil

If the chicken or turkey is not precooked, cook it first in a separate pan. Preheat the oven to 450° F. Pour in the egg whites or Egg Beaters into a skillet and cook over medium heat for a minute or so. Mix in the vegetables together with the meat and the oil and cook until the eggs are as you like them. Remove from heat. Put an ounce of mozzarella on top of the omelet. Put the skillet in the oven and bake for several minutes until the cheese is lightly brown.

Serves two
Calories—200 each

Amen Centers Rainbow Omelet

2 cups raw fresh spinach
1 cup raw fresh broccoli
½ each red and yellow peppers
garlic powder
extra-virgin olive oil
4 eggs (DHA enhanced)
½ small avocado, sliced
1 oz. mozzarella cheese, shredded

Preheat the oven to 450° F. Sauté the vegetables (do the spinach separately) in a small amount of olive oil. Add garlic powder. Whisk the eggs together and pour into an oven-ready heated skillet over medium heat. As the eggs become slightly firm, place the vegetables on top, add the sliced avocado, then sprinkle on the cheese. Remove from heat. Put skillet in the oven and bake the omelet for several minutes until the cheese is lightly brown.

Serves two
Calories—375 each

Red, White, and Blue Smoothie

½ to ¾ cup plain yogurt
2 tbsp. flax oil
1 tsp. Stevia or Splenda (a natural sweetener)
½ Gala or Washington apple
¼ cup frozen strawberries
1 cup frozen blueberries

Mix ingredients in blender. Serve chilled.

Serves two
Calories—250 each

LUNCH RECIPES

Spinach Salad

2 cups fresh spinach
handful of walnuts
3 strawberries, sliced

1 hard-boiled egg, sliced
3 oz. turkey breast
½ avocado, sliced
2 tbsp. Paul Newman Low Calorie Balsamic Vinaigrette Dressing

Mix ingredients and serve.

Serves one
Calories—425

Newport Beach Blueberry Chicken Salad

3 oz. chicken breast
2 cups mixed baby greens
5 cherry tomatoes
½ red bell pepper
handful fresh blueberries
2 tbsp. extra-virgin olive oil
3 tbsp. freshly squeezed lemon juice
pinch of fresh garlic

Serves one
Calories—275

Green and Wild

3 oz. of Alaskan Wild Salmon
lemon pepper, to taste
salt, to taste
4 oz. cooked spinach
1 tbsp. olive oil

Grill salmon on barbecue with spices. Sauté spinach in olive oil. Serve together.

Serves one
Calories—300

Veggie Sandwich

2 slices whole wheat bread
1 slice Jack cheese, cut in 4 pieces

3–4 spinach leaves
½ tomato, sliced
1 mild green chili, sliced
½ red bell pepper, julienned
¼ cucumber, sliced

Put cheese and veggies on bread slices. Grill in George Foreman grill 4 or 5 minutes. Serve with cucumber garnish.

Serves one
Calories—350

DINNER

Italian Tomatoes and Pork Chops

2 lean pork chops, fat cut away
salt, pepper, and garlic powder
1 14-oz. can S&W Italian stewed tomatoes
½ cup fresh mushrooms, sliced

Sprinkle the pork chops with salt, pepper, and garlic. Place them on top of the stewed tomatoes and mushrooms in a covered skillet on the stove and cook until done. It is amazing!

Serves one
Calories—approximately 400

JT's Grilled Salmon or Trout

1 3-oz. filet salmon or trout
lemon slices
½ red and yellow pepper
onions, to taste
lemon pepper
salt

Put the fish on top of the vegetables on a piece of foil. Wrap loosely, and make a short tent to seal it. Place on barbecue or in oven and cook until done, about 20 minutes.

Serves one
Calories—200

Dorie's Truly Amazing Lamb, Beans, and Rice

½ cup Mahatma long-grain rice
¼ tsp. salt
¼ tsp. pepper
½ tsp. cinnamon
12 oz. lean lamb (all fat cut away), chopped
½ small onion, chopped
28 oz. diced tomatoes
¼ tsp. pepper
2 cups fresh green beans
1 oz. feta cheese
1 tbsp. olive oil

Place rice in 1 cup boiling water with salt, pepper, and cinnamon. Cook till tender. Sauté lamb and onion in olive oil till brown. Add diced tomatoes and pepper. Simmer about 15 minutes. Add green beans and simmer 5 minutes more. Serve lamb and beans over rice. Top with feta cheese.

Serves four
Calories per serving—about 450

DESSERTS

EZ Blue Rider

8 oz. frozen blueberries
6 oz. Greek-style yogurt
1 tsp. vanilla (can help raise serotonin levels)
cinnamon, to taste (an antioxidant that balances blood sugar)

Let the blueberries thaw for 20 minutes. Stir them into the yogurt and vanilla. Sprinkle with cinnamon.

Serves one
Calories—200

EZ Blueberry Ice Cream (the teens in my house go nuts for this one)

8 oz. frozen blueberries
4 tbsp. heavy cream
touch of Stevia (a natural sweetener)

Mix ingredients in a blender, then serve.

Serves one
Calories—260
(about the same as a Snickers bar,
but much healthier and tastier)

SNACK

Homemade Turkey Jerky (this is my personal favorite, and I eat it all the time while writing)

Take raw turkey breasts, and slice them thinly with the grain. Put a little salt, pepper, and garlic powder on the meat. Put it in a dehydrator. It's cheap, very tasty, and the kids like it a lot.

EATING OUT

Given the fast pace of most of our lives, many people (including me) eat in fast-food restaurants. I am fortunate to live in California, where we have El Pollo Loco (suits a psychiatrist), where it is easy to find balanced, healthful meals. Due to customer demand, most fast-food restaurants also have healthier alternatives. For a fast-food breakfast, I often have a combination of scrambled eggs and a piece of fruit from McDonald's. For lunch or dinner there are many choices. The Wendy's large-size chili (no fries, saltines, or Coke) is only 300 calories and is a good balance between carbohydrates, proteins, and fats. Jack in the Box's chicken fajita pita (hold the onion rings and soft drink) is also 300 calories and is nicely balanced. Burger King's BK Broiler, minus a quarter of the bun, also fits this category. At Subway a turkey breast sub with extra meat helps make a balanced meal (no cookie, of course). They also have a great low-carb wrap sandwich to which you can add a variety of veggies. I am very fond of the new salads at most fast-food restaurants. Some of them are quite tasty and very low in calories, but be careful with the salad dressings, as they often have more calories than the salads themselves.

LET'S GO SHOPPING THROUGH THE MARKET

I grew up in grocery stores. My father owns a grocery chain in southern California, and I have spent my life in and out of them. Many people get confused about how to shop in a brain-healthy way. So here are some tips.

1. Stay away from foods at the checkout stand. They are impulse foods (geared to people with low frontal lobes), such as candy and soft drinks, and grocers hope to add to your bill by getting you to buy them before you leave.

2. Shop on the outside aisles of the store. You will find the produce department, meat and fish department, and dairy departments on the outside aisles. It's best if most of your food comes from there.

3. Bring a list, and stick to it. Planning ahead of time will get you in and out with what you need and help you avoid impulse buying.

4. Do not shop when you are hungry! You will buy more food, and more junk food, than you need.

5. Buy in bulk when possible. I buy twenty to forty packages of frozen blueberries at a time. The checkout clerks often look at me in a strange way. I always tell them about brain berries.

6. In the produce department go for the spinach, broccoli, red peppers, oranges, lemons, and limes.

7. In the meat department get skinless chicken and turkey, salmon, and ahi tuna. In my fast-paced lifestyle, I often buy a roasted chicken (very tender) and cut it up to put in omelets and on salads throughout the week.

8. In the dairy case look for plain yogurt and soymilk, DHA eggs, or Egg Beaters.

9. In the deli case look for low-fat cheeses, such as mozzarella and string cheese. Choose lean meats, such as Canadian bacon.

10. In the frozen-food section look for frozen fruits and vegetables. I already mentioned the blueberries. Stir-fry vegetables are often low in calories and have many of the foods we want with no preservatives.

11. Stay away from store-bought fruit juices. Many people, especially parents, have the mistaken idea that they are health foods, but they are mainly liquid sugar with a few vitamins added. Whole fruit is much better, or the pulp-filled juices you squeeze at home.

12. There is no constitutional amendment that children have a right to junk food. Parents somehow feel that they are depriving their kids if they are not allowed to have cookies and ice cream. Teach them how

to eat for their brains when they are young, and they are likely to develop good habits that will serve them their whole lives. Exposure equals preference, so what you feed them now can help determine their long-term food choices.

At work I do not allow employees to have candy on their desks. It invites sharing—not only the candy but also the low blood sugar, the foggy minds, and the lower productivity that come from the candy. What businesses serve at meetings is silly. If they understood about eating for the brain, they would lose the coffee, juices, muffins, Danishes, and doughnuts and replace them with water, herbal teas, fruit, cheeses, whole grains, deviled eggs, and nuts.

Recently the Amen Clinics had a company board meeting. Here was the menu, seeking to honor healthy brains.

- Spinach Salad, with red peppers, tomatoes, and an olive oil vinaigrette
- JT's Grilled Salmon and Trout
- Steamed broccoli and asparagus
- EZ Blue Rider (for dessert)

One final thought on food. Your thoughts about and attitude toward food will either help you create a better brain or throw you off track. But it is easy to stay the course if you see this nutritional plan as not only good for you but an advantage for your brain and body. If you feel deprived or have a negative attitude about it, there is no way you'll stick to it.

BRAIN WORKOUTS

KEEPING THE BRAIN YOUNG THROUGH MENTAL EXERCISE

"We must CHALLENGE the brain. It gets bored; we know that well."
—Marian Diamond

"You know you've got to exercise your brain just like your muscles."
—Will Rogers

Your brain is like a muscle: the more you use it, the more you can continue using it. New learning causes new connections to form in the brain. No learning causes the brain to start disconnecting itself. No matter what your age, mental exercise has a global, positive effect on your brain.

In three decades of brain research, celebrated neuroscientist Marian Diamond, of the University of California at Berkeley, has helped revolutionize the way we think about brain health. In a lecture to the American Society on Aging in 2001 she said, "We now know that with proper stimulation and an enriched environment, the human brain can continue to develop at any age." Her work used middle-aged rats, the equivalent of sixty-year-old humans, and older rats, some corresponding to humans at ninety. Dr. Diamond and her co-workers were able to show that with added enrichment—such as colorful toys and balls, exercise equipment, new mazes, and other rodents for companionship—the size and cognitive ability of the rats' brains improved. Rats that were raised in social groups and had a changing variety of toys and other experiences were much better at running mazes than were rats reared in isolation and deprived of stimulation. Their brains also looked different. They had many more sprouting dendrites, nerve cells, and blood vessels and a thicker cerebral cortex. "We used middle-aged rats partly because they have a similar cortex to humans," Diamond said. Diamond, in her early seventies, says it was "comforting to find we can change the brain at any age. We're saying that if you use your brain, you can change it as much as a younger brain." She said it may take the older brain longer to respond, but change does happen. In her opinion, people would be wise to think of their brain as a muscle. Left in isolation, evidence shows, brain cells begin to shrink and shut down.

The best mental exercise is acquiring new knowledge and doing things that you have not done before. New learning helps the brain. Doing the things you have always done is not helpful for the brain, even if those things are fairly complicated. For instance, I have spent many hours over the past fifteen years reading brain scans. When I first started reading them in 1991, it took me a lot of time and mental effort. My brain worked hard to read them correctly. Over the years, as my brain has become more and more familiar with the scans and the technology that underlies them, reading a scan takes much less time and mental effort. If all I did from here on out was read scans and not engage in other forms of novel learning, my brain would no longer benefit from the work. Whenever the brain does something over and over, even a complicated task, it learns how to do it using less and less energy. Learning a new medical technique, a new hobby, or a new game helps establish new connections, thus maintaining and improving the function of other less-often-used brain areas.

The famous Nuns Study, conducted by researchers at the Rush University Medical Center in Chicago, shows the power of this "use it or lose it" principle of mental exercise. The researchers studied how often 801 older nuns, priests, and other clergy engaged in mentally stimulating activities, such as reading a newspaper, over five years. They discovered that those who increased their mental activity over the five years reduced their chance of developing Alzheimer's disease by one-third. These more mentally active individuals also reduced their age-related decline in overall mental abilities by 50 percent, in concentration and attention span by 60 percent, and in mental processing speed by 30 percent.

Learning has a very real effect on neurons: it keeps them firing and makes it easier for them to fire. The brain has approximately a thousand trillion synapses, each one of which may wither and die if it is not actively firing. Like muscles that don't get used, idle nerve cells waste away. The brain has many, many different circuits. Any set of circuits that does not get used grows weak. For example, middle-aged people who go back to college often feel slow and stupid at first, but after a few semesters of mental exercise, they find academic studies easy again. With age, the level of activity of the enzymes in one's cells starts to decline. The cells become less efficient, and the brain isn't quite as agile as that of an eighteen-year-old. But in some ways younger people are at a disadvantage. In certain respects the fifty-year-old will do better in academic studies, because as one ages one's frontal lobes are better developed, which usually helps a person pay better attention in class and ask better questions. A more developed frontal lobe allows you to take better advantage of new knowledge, to know what to focus on, and to relate it to life experiences so that it has more useful value to you. The eighteen-year-old may be able to memorize facts more easily, but his frontal lobe isn't as good at selecting *which* facts to memorize.

The human brain depends on proper stimulation, such as from reading, to grow and develop in healthy ways throughout childhood and to maintain its functioning into old age. When you stimulate neurons in the right way, you make them more efficient; they function better, and you are more likely to have an active, learning brain throughout your life. Long-term potentiation (LTP) is the physiology of learning. It is the process of invigorating (or potentiating) neurons to do their job over a long period of time. Learning is accomplished, quite simply, through the repetition of an act that causes actual physical changes in neurons and their synapses. LTP causes the nerve endings to get bigger, which creates a significant advantage on three fronts. One, they are harder to damage. Two, the larger surface area on the neurons allows for greater signals to pass between cells, enhancing efficient communication. And three, in the process of potentiation, receiving neurons can generate their own signals with less input in the future; this means that once LTP has occurred, it takes less energy to do something well. For instance, a pianist who has been practicing a piece by Rachmaninoff will be able, after a year, to play it without struggle, without thinking about it, because he has been steadily stimulating the synapses in the neurons that control his finger movements so they can execute the proper sequence to play the piece. He has "potentiated" his neurons in just the right way to accomplish that goal. In order to keep learning, he must begin work on a new piece.

THIRTEEN PRACTICAL WAYS TO EXERCISE YOUR BRAIN

1. Dedicate yourself to new learning. Put fifteen minutes in your day into learning something new. Einstein said that if someone spent fifteen minutes a day learning something new, in a year he would be an expert. As in school or business, commitment is critical to achieving greatness—or a great brain.

2. Take a class about something new and interesting. In many areas of the country community colleges and groups such as the Learning Annex (www.learningannex.com) offer low-cost classes on a wide variety of subjects. Attend a new class on a subject totally unrelated to your day-to-day life. It is important to challenge your brain to learn new and novel things. Examples include square dancing (great exercise), chess, tai chi, yoga, or sculpture. Working with modeling clay or Play-Doh can be good for both children and adults to help them grow new connections. It helps develop agility and hand-brain coordination.

3. Cross-train at work. Learn someone else's job. Maybe even switch jobs for several weeks. This benefits the business and employees alike, as both workers will develop new skills and better brain function. For example, in a grocery store employees can be taught to work as checkout clerks, stock shelves, order products, and alternately work in the produce, grocery, and dairy sections of the store.

4. Improve your skills at things you already do. Some repetitive mental stimulation is okay, as long as you look to expand your skill and knowledge base. Common activities such as gardening, sewing, playing bridge, reading, painting, and doing crossword puzzles have value, but push yourself to do different gardening techniques, more complex sewing patterns, play bridge against more talented players, read new authors on varied subjects, learn a new painting technique, and work harder at crossword puzzles. Pushing your brain to new heights helps to keep it healthy and strong.

5. Limit television for kids and adults. A study published in the journal *Pediatrics* reported that for every hour a day children watch TV, there is a 10 percent increased chance that they will be diagnosed with ADD. This means that if children watch five hours a day, they have a 50 percent chance of being diagnosed with ADD. According to the American Academy of Child and

Adolescent Psychiatry, children spend three to four hours a day watching TV. Another study, and several others like it, showed that increased television watching in childhood put people at risk for problems as adults. Dr. R. J. Hancox and colleagues from the department of preventive and social medicine in Dunedin, New Zealand, assessed approximately a thousand children born in 1972–73, at regular intervals up to age twenty-six. They found a significant association between higher body-mass index, lower physical fitness, increased cigarette smoking, and raised serum cholesterol. All these factors are involved in brain illnesses, such as strokes or Alzheimer's disease. Yet another study found that adults who watched TV two or more hours a day had a significantly higher risk of Alzheimer's disease. Watching TV is usually a "no-brain" activity. To be fair, these studies did not specify if watching programs that teach you something have the same effect as situation comedies or sports. I suspect that no-brain TV shows are the primary problem.

6. Limit video games. As a child psychiatrist and a father of three children, I have thought a lot about video games over the past fifteen years. At first, I found them great fun to play. Then I started to worry. Action video games have been studied using brain-imaging techniques that look at blood flow and activity patterns. Video games have been found to work in the basal ganglia, one of the pleasure centers in the brain (see Chapter 5). In fact, this is the same part of the brain that lights up when researchers inject a person with cocaine. My experience with patients and one of my own children is that they tend to get hooked on the games and play so much that it can deteriorate their schoolwork, their work, and their social time, a bit like a drug. Some children and adults actually do get hooked on them.

Some scientific literature reports that video games may increase the frequency of seizures in people who are sensitive to them. You may remember the seizure scare on December 16, 1997, when the Japanese cartoon "Pocket Monster" (Pokémon) showed an explosion of red, white, and yellow lights that triggered 730 Japanese children in one evening to go to the hospital with new-onset seizures. The condition is called photosensitive seizures (seizures triggered by light). I often think video games trigger subclinical seizures in vulnerable kids and adults, causing behavior or learning problems.

Two studies from the University of Missouri examined the effects of violent video games (a significant percentage of video games) on aggression. One study found that violent real-life simulation video-game play was positively related to aggressive behavior and delinquency. The more people played, the more trouble they seemed to have. Academic performance deteriorated with increased time spent playing video games. In the second study, laboratory exposure to a graphically violent video game increased aggressive thoughts and behavior. The results from both studies suggest that exposure to violent video games will increase aggressive behavior in both the short term (such as laboratory aggression) and the long term (such as delinquency). A comprehensive review of other studies found time and again that exposure to violent video games is significantly linked to increases in aggressive behavior, aggressive thoughts, aggressive feelings, and cardiovascular arousal, and to decreases in helping behavior. None of this is good for overall brain health.

I recently had an experience that highlights how important TV and video games are to mental health problems. Joshua, a twelve-year-old boy, had been seeing me for several years for aggression, oppositional behavior, moodiness, and school failure. It took me quite a while to get him stabilized, but with parent training, psychotherapy, and some supplements, he was doing great. Then he went to stay with his dad for three weeks and totally relapsed. His father let him watch all the TV and play all the video games he wanted. Joshua quickly reverted back to his nasty behavior and actually started to pull out his own hair (a sign of anxiety and compulsiveness). When we stopped both TV and video games, he quickly improved.

When video games came into my home, my son was in the sixth grade (fifteen years ago). I noticed over time that he played more and more, even when he was told to stop. His grades went down, and his level of defiance went up. After two years of difficult behavior, I took the games out of the house. Thankfully, my girls have never been very interested. I do not think video games give kids or adults any long-term value. They do not help you get most jobs (one exception may be flight-simulator games), and I think they train the brain to need more and more stimulation to be able to focus. There are many reasons why the incidence in learning and behavior problems has doubled in the last twenty years. I believe video games may be part of the puzzle.

7. Join a reading group that keeps you accountable to new learning.
Almost any mental activity you enjoy can be used to protect your brain. The essential requirement is that it activates several different brain areas, one of which should be the hippocampus (in the temporal lobes), which stores new information for retrieval later on. By recalling information (using your hip-

pocampus), you are protecting your brain's memory centers. In essence, as long as you learn something new and work to recall it later for discussions, you are protecting your short-term memory.

Reading stimulates a wide variety of brain areas that process, understand, and analyze what you read, then store it for later recall if you decide it's worth remembering. The neurons in these activated brain areas are stimulated with specific patterns of information. Each time you read, the neurons activated in your brain's visual circuits further strengthen their synapses so you can process what you read with increasing efficiency. Each time you try to understand what you read, the neurons in your working memory circuits strengthen their synapses so you can understand reading material with increasing efficiency. Each time you try to learn something you read for recall later, the neurons in the hippocampus further strengthen their synapses so you can encode and store new information with increasing efficiency. Each time you try and recall what you just learned, after a delay of at least two minutes, neurons in the frontal lobe further strengthen their synapses so you can retrieve stored information with increasing efficiency. Given this information, it is even better to join a reading group, where you are pushed to remember what you read for later discussion, than to read novels or newspapers that you may just forget.

8. Practice does not make perfect. Perfect practice make perfect. The brain does not interpret what you feed into it; it simply translates it. When you are learning to play the piano, the brain doesn't care if you are becoming a great piano player or a terrible piano player. Consequently, if you repeat imperfect fingering, you will become very good at playing imperfectly. If you are training yourself to be a perfect pianist, it is essential that you practice perfectly and not learn bad habits or sloppy fingering of the keys. To play well, it is helpful to work with a professional who can correct your mistakes. Your brain doesn't care what you give it, so if you care whether you do something well or badly, you must be certain that you are giving your brain the right training. This is why it is essential that children have good teachers who watch and monitor their progress, and why we need to have effective training programs in the workplace. Teaching someone to do something well at the start prevents them from developing bad habits, which get solidified in the brain and are subsequently hard to retrain.

I was once a consultant to a large medical practice that had significant employee turnover problems. As I investigated the problem, I discovered that the office manager was poorly trained and had little social skill. She was rude and inappropriate with patients, and she subsequently modeled that behavior to the front office staff. She was resistant to retraining (a cingulate gyrus that likely worked too hard), and ultimately she needed to be replaced.

Effective initial training in the workplace and in school is essential to developing effective, happy employees and students. We do not just train people, we train brains.

9. Break the routine of your life to stimulate new parts of your brain. To activate the other side of your brain and gain access to both hemispheres, do the opposite of what feels natural. Write with your other hand, shoot basketballs with both hands, hit baseballs left-handed (if you are right-handed), play table tennis left-handed, shoot a rifle sighting with your other eye, use the mouse with your other hand—make your brain feel uncomfortable. In essence, break the patterned routine in your life to challenge your brain to make new connections. Here are some more ideas.

- Make love in a different way.
- Try a sport you've never tried before.
- Take a class in a subject you know nothing about.
- Learn new cooking recipes.
- Do some volunteer work—see how good you'll feel when you help others.
- Try a different shampoo/soap/shaving cream/razor/toothpaste/perfume/cologne.
- Go to church, or a different church.
- Go to an opera or symphony concert.
- Join a self-development group.
- Spend time reading the dictionary or a reference book—learn a new word each day.
- Take time out each day to strengthen a special relationship, with a spouse, lover, child, or friend.
- Make a new friend—call up someone and ask him or her to do something with you.
- Contact an old friend you haven't talked to in a while.
- Submit a new idea at work, maybe even one you've thought about for a while but were too embarrassed to mention because you thought no one would be interested in it.

• Forgive someone you hold a grudge against. This is a new activity for many people.

10. *Compare how similar things work.* Evaluating similar items—how different pitchers throw a curve ball, the many ways painters can paint ocean scenes, the varying spices in meals—gives your brain a sensory workout. Looking at similarities and differences helps the brain's ability to think abstractly and challenges our frontal lobes. Learning to see, hear, feel, or taste subtle changes will enhance your sensory ability and stimulate brain growth.

11. *Visit new and different places.* Traveling to new and interesting places helps the brain by exposing it to new experiences, scents, sights, and people. Using maps stimulates the brain in new and different ways and also exercises our parietal lobes, which are responsible for visual-spatial guidance.

12. *Cultivate smart friends.* People are contagious. You become like the people with whom you spend time. Work on developing friendships with new, interesting people. You can trade ideas, get new perspectives, and generally stretch your mind if you are surrounded by fascinating folks. In playing any game, if you want to be better, you have to play with people who are better than you, to push you to your limit. The same principle holds true in pushing your brain to new heights. Spend time with people who challenge you.

13. *Treat learning problems to help kids and adults stay in school.* Numerous studies show that better-educated people have less risk of Alzheimer's disease and cognitive decline. Millions of children, teens, and adults suffer from ADD and learning problems that cause them to struggle in school or with learning despite having normal or even high intelligence. Recognizing these problems and getting them the help they need is essential to making lifelong learning a reality. You can take an online test for ADD at www. amenclinic.com.

Mental exercise is as important as diet and physical exercise for keeping both your body and brain strong.

13

EXERCISE FOR YOUR BRAIN

Physical exercise protects and enhances your brain. It is perhaps the single most important thing you can do to keep your neurons healthy over time. Moderate exercise improves the heart's ability to pump blood throughout the body and helps maintain healthy blood flow to the brain, which increases oxygen and glucose delivery. Exercise also reduces damage to neurons from toxic substances from the environment and enhances insulin's ability to prevent high-blood-sugar levels, thereby reducing the risk of diabetes. Physical exercise also helps protect the short-term memory structures in your temporal lobes (hippocampus) from high-stress conditions. Stress causes the adrenal glands to produce excessive amounts of the hormone cortisol, which has been found to kill cells in the hippocampus and hurt memory. In fact, people with Alzheimer's disease have higher cortisol levels than normal aging people.

Physical exercise makes the whole body healthier. It does this by improving the tone of the blood vessels, which decreases the risk for high blood pressure, stroke, and heart disease and increases blood flow to every organ in the body to make them hardier. Additionally, it helps maintain coordination, agility, and speed. The Honolulu Study of Aging found that untreated high blood pressure during midlife (forty to sixty years old) greatly increases the risk for dementia. For middle-aged people with a systolic blood pressure of 160 mm Hg or higher, or a diastolic blood pressure of 90 mm Hg or higher, the risk of dementia after seventy years old was 3.8 to 4.8 times greater than those whose high blood pressure was treated. This study emphasizes the importance of getting regular exercise and proper treatment for any medical conditions you may have.

Exercise actually stimulates neurogenesis, the ability of the brain to generate new neurons. When laboratory rats exercise, research shows, they generate new neurons in the frontal lobe and hippocampus, which survive for about four weeks and then die off unless they are stimulated. If you stimulate these new neurons through mental or social interaction, they connect to other neurons and become integrated into brain circuits that help maintain their functions throughout your life. This is why people who *only* work out at the gym are not as smart as people who work out and then go to the library. Exercise exerts a protective effect on hippocampal neurons that lasts about three days. Therefore the minimum frequency of exercise is every three days, or three times a week. Studies have shown that the more frequently you exercise, the greater the benefits.

Lack of exercise negatively affects blood supply in the body. Exercise increases the chemical nitric oxide, which helps keep blood vessel walls open and round. In order to keep your blood vessels open, blood must pulse through them. Without good blood flow, the levels of nitric oxide drop and cause the blood vessel walls to become distorted and limit the flow of blood. The most effective way to make blood flow pulse through arteries is to exercise. Without pulsatile flow, the blood vessels in the deep areas of the brain distort and limit blood flow, increasing the chance of tiny strokes. Over a period of years, these strokes accumulate and cause these deep brain areas to stop working. The deep brain areas control leg movement, coordinated body movement, and speed of thinking and behaving. Strokes in these areas produce a clinical picture that closely resembles Parkinson's disease because it affects similar brain areas. This is why people who do not exercise after forty years of age are not as mentally sharp as people who exercise regularly.

Developing a regular habit of physical exercise is a major preventive strategy for age-related memory problems, but don't wait until you're seventy-five to start exercising. The Sydney Older Persons Study found that exercise levels in persons seventy-five years and older did not reduce risk of Alzheimer's disease or other causes of dementia. This means that it is important to establish a regular habit of exercise in your life now, not to wait until your seventies to start.

Exercise also enhances the production of glutathione, which is the major antioxidant in all cells, to protect your muscles and other tissues against free radical damage. Conversely, chronic inactivity ("couch potato" syndrome) reduces cell glutathione levels, so that free radicals can damage your cells and trigger programmed cell death.

Research has shown that the benefits of mild to moderate exercise include:

- Protecting brain cells against toxins, including free radicals
- Repairing cellular DNA to help protect against programmed cell death
- Reducing the risks of cognitive impairment and dementia due to Alzheimer's disease by about 50 percent in persons over sixty-five
- Preserving mental abilities after age seventy
- Reducing the risks of heart disease and stroke by improving cholesterol and fat metabolism, plus improving blood, oxygen, and glucose delivery to tissues
- Reducing the risk of diabetes by making insulin better control your blood sugar (glucose) and increasing your lean-to-fat mass ratio
- Reducing the risk of osteoporosis by reducing bone loss (estrogen enhances this effect)
- Reducing the risk of depression
- Reducing the risks of colon and breast cancer
- Reducing the risks of falling by improving muscle tone and endurance, and reducing strokes to the deep brain areas

In a large study from Quebec, Dr. D. Laurin and colleagues explored the association between physical activity and the risk of cognitive impairment and dementia. They gathered information from a community sample of 9,008 randomly selected men and women sixty-five or older who were evaluated in the 1991–92 Canadian Study of Health and Aging, a prospective group study of dementia. Of the 6,434 eligible subjects who were cognitively normal at baseline, 4,615 completed a five-year follow-up. Screening and clinical evaluations were done at both times of the study. In 1996–97, 3,894 subjects remained without cognitive impairment, 436 were diagnosed as having cognitive impairment but no dementia (mild cognitive impairment), and 285 were diagnosed as having dementia. Compared with lack of exercise, physical activity was associated with lower risks of cognitive impairment, Alzheimer's disease, and dementia of any type. High levels of physical activity were associated with even more reduced risks. They concluded that regular physical activity could represent an important and potent protective factor against cognitive decline and dementia in elderly people.

The best kinds of exercise improve the pump force of your heart (cardiovascular exercise) and strengthen the muscles of your body (resistive exercise). Cardiovascular exercise involves gradually warming up your muscles, then exercising them for thirty minutes or more (by walking, running, swimming, rowing, cycling, stair climbing, cross-country skiing, and so on), to develop muscle tone for endurance. Resistive exercise builds muscle strength by exercising the muscles against resistance (by doing sit-ups, push-ups, lifting weights, rowing, stair climbing, swimming, cycling, cross-country skiing, and so on). As you can see, several types of exercise fall into both categories, including rowing, stair climbing, swimming, cycling, and cross-country skiing. You can also make walking and running into resistive exercises if you add weights.

TABLE TENNIS IS THE WORLD'S BEST BRAIN SPORT

My favorite exercise is table tennis. Some people laugh when I say this at lectures, but I am very serious. "Ping-Pong," they scoff, "is only a basement recreational game." You certainly haven't met my mother (the mother with the perfect brain). I remember when I was a young child and would sit in the backyard, amazed that she would beat all comers to the table. She was intense and had wonderful reflexes. I remember watching her trying to keep up with the little white ball. I played a lot as a child with my siblings, but I didn't really become skilled until I spent three years in Germany as a young soldier in the U.S. Army. The military, as highlighted in the movie *Forrest Gump*, has tennis tables in almost all recreation centers. With my childhood background, I was better than most players and won several tournaments. I then developed a friendship with a soldier from the West Indies, René, who was a championship-caliber player. We spent hour after hour playing at the USO in Frankfurt. One of my strategies in life is to try to be with people who are better than me at whatever I am doing. They help me be better, and losing to René was no big deal as long as I kept getting better. I was thrilled that at the end of my tour I was finally able to beat him. We joined a German table tennis club and spent many hours interacting with our new friends around the table.

If you are an American, you still may think that calling table tennis a sport is silly, but I think it is the best brain sport ever. It is highly aerobic, uses both the upper and lower body, is great for eye-hand coordination and reflexes, and causes you to use many different areas of the brain at once as you are tracking the ball, planning shots and strategies, and figuring out spins. It is like aerobic chess. Plus, it causes very few head injuries. Table tennis—or Ping-Pong, the name given to the sport by the Parker Brothers game company to sell more equipment—is the second most popular organized sport in the world. Even more impressive, it is the youngest of the world's major sports. At the competitive level, players hit the ball in excess of ninety miles per hour across the table!

Table tennis is now recognized as an Olympic sport, making its debut in the 1988 Seoul games. You can find the sport televised throughout the world at any given time. From the Hong Kong Invitational to the World Table Tennis Championships to the Olympics, table tennis is completely sold out for all sessions.

In the United States there are many table tennis clubs and even more great players. The best way to start playing table tennis is to get a table and learn the basics of the game. I often recommend getting a USATT (United States of America Table Tennis) coach to ramp up skill quickly. The game is more fun if you can play well. You can learn more about table tennis rules, equipment, coaches, and places to play at www.usatt.org.

Exercise has profound and broad-based effects on health. A study done at Case Western Reserve University looked at how much TV people watch each day, which correlates with their exercise level. People who watched two or more hours of TV a day (couch potatoes) were twice as likely to develop Alzheimer's. In contrast, people over forty years old who exercise at least thirty minutes per session two or more times a week reaped many benefits.

The data on exercise is impressive and incontrovertible. Our distant ancestors exercised as part of daily life when they hunted and gathered food, fled their enemies, and tracked down a mate. In the modern world, where we sit in a cubicle in front of a computer screen all day, then come home at night and slump in a recliner to watch TV, we have to make an effort to do what our ancestors did as a matter of course. Our bodies did not evolve to be motionless and inert; they evolved with muscles, hearts, and cardiovascular systems that need to be activated.

The greatest obstacle most people have in committing to regular exercise is making it a habit. People don't think twice about brushing their teeth, showering, or dressing in the morning, or adjusting the rearview mirror when they climb into the car, because these activities are all habits that they've trained their brains to perform automatically. A habit is a series of actions your brain executes, when you tell it to do so, fairly automatically and without effort. But it requires many repetitions before your brain learns to automatically perform a function. Think of how many times it took you to learn to ride your bike without training wheels. The real challenge of exercise is to train your brain to make exercise a habit.

The best chance of making exercise a habit is to schedule a specific time and place to exercise each day or at least on specific days each week. Consider using the same shoes and clothing and doing the workout in the same place, but have a variety of exercises to choose from so you can vary the routine. The idea is to exercise consistently according to schedule for the first few months. After several months you will find that you no longer think about whether you want to get out there and work out or not—you just do it. When you reach that point, it has become a habit, one that will keep you and your brain healthy and that will save you more money than any other single thing you will ever do for your health. It's well worth the effort.

COORDINATE YOUR BRAIN

Coordination enhancement, like exercise, helps balance brain function. The brain's major coordination center is thought to be the cerebellum, about the size of a fist, located at the back bottom of the brain. It is involved in balance, posture, gait, and motor coordination. In addition, it is thought to be part of thought coordination, or how quickly you can integrate new information and think on your feet. Given that the cerebellum has about half of all the brain's neurons, it may also be involved in processing speed, much like the Pentium chips running our newer computers.

If you are as old as I am—fifty, at the time I am writing this book—you may remember the old AT and XT processing chips in the computers of the early 1980s. They were amazing at the time, but compared to the computers of today, they were ever so slow. I remember trying to pull up image files on the old computers. Sometimes they would take twenty or thirty minutes to upload. The image would come up one line at a time. And remember the early days of very slow Internet modem connections? It would take so long to go to a new site or download material that you could get a cup of tea and read the paper. Having a small or sluggish cerebellum is like living in a Pentium world with an old XT computer in your head; you are slower, have less processing speed, and are more easily frustrated. In fact, problems in the cerebellum are associated with slow movements, slowed speech, and slowed thought processes.

My patient Ralph's case clearly illustrates the functions of the cerebellum and what happens when things go wrong. Ralph was sent to me by his neurologist because he was having family problems; he was often socially inappropriate and was argumentative and uncooperative. As a child he had had a viral brain infection that left him with a permanent inability to perform co-ordinated movements, speak clearly, and behave appropriately at work or in social circumstances. He had been fired from many jobs because of this "attitude" problem. Despite being intelligent, he also had problems with learning and memory. His SPECT scan showed virtually no activity in his cerebellum—damage from the viral attack when he was young. At the time of the scan his speech was slow, his thought processes were delayed, it took him almost a minute to answer questions, and his walk was slow and unsteady. After treating him for three months with memantine (a new medication for memory loss) and targeted exercises, the family reported that he was more coordinated, spoke more clearly, and behaved more appropriately. Soon he was able to start working again.

After doing research on our database, we found highly statistical relationships between low cerebellar activity and the following issues:

- Poor planning skills
- Absence of clear goals or forward thinking
- Inattention to detail
- Difficulty expressing empathy for others
- Trouble maintaining an organized work or living area
- Messy room and/or multiple piles around room
- Poor or messy handwriting
- Messy or disorganized notebook/paperwork
- Frequent lateness or rushing
- Not writing down assignments or tasks and forgetting what to do
- Light sensitivity, irritation from glare, sunlight, headlights, or streetlights
- Feeling of tension, tiredness, sleepiness, or headaches with reading
- Problems judging distance and difficulty with escalators, stairs, ball sports, or driving
- Greater sensitivity to the environment than others
- Greater sensitivity to noise than others
- Particular sensitivity to touch or to certain clothing or clothing tags
- Unusual sensitivity to certain smells
- Sensitivity to movement or craving for spinning activities
- Tendency to be clumsy or accident-prone

According to our database, people's main struggles with low activity in the cerebellum appear to be centered on planning, goal-setting, details, organization, time management, perception, coordination, and filtering out extraneous input. Interestingly, alcohol intoxication affects all of these areas—clumsiness, bad judgment, disorganized behavior, altered perceptions—and has been found to be directly toxic to cells in the cerebellum. The scans of our alcoholics tend to show very low activity in this part of the brain. *Clue number one to enhancing cerebellar activity—reduce alcohol consumption.*

The next step to optimizing cerebellar function and cognitive speed and agility is engaging in regular exercises that activate this coordination center. Activating the cerebellum helps it work more efficiently and with greater speed. In our scans, professional athletes and musicians (not the drug-affected ones) show the best cerebellar activity. They dedicate their lives to using coordinated body efforts to perform their skills. The ongoing repetition of coordinated activities (practice) dramatically helps this part of the brain. The average person who wishes to make use of this principle needs to put coordination exercises into his or her weekly routine. Any exercise that enhances fine or gross motor coordination can be helpful, such as playing a musical instrument, learning or practicing a sport that requires skill (with little risk of a brain injury, such as golf, tennis, or table tennis), doing martial arts or yoga, and dancing.

Juggling may be a particularly good exercise for the brain. When people spend three months learning to juggle, according to a paper published in *Nature,* parts of their brains grow. Researchers in Germany split twenty-four students into two groups, one of which was given three months to learn a classic three-ball cascade juggling routine. Brain scans were then carried out on both sets of volunteers. The brains of the jugglers and nonjugglers were scanned before and after the three-month learning period. The jugglers had more gray matter in the temporal and parietal lobes. The study indicates that the brain can grow and become stronger based on what we do and practice. A cool website to learn to juggle is www.juggling.org.

There are also structured programs geared toward enhancing cerebellar activity. Two of these programs are the Interactive Metronome and the Brain Gym.

The **Interactive Metronome** (IM) combines the concept of a musical metronome with a computer program that measures, assesses, and improves a person's rhythm and timing. It helps the brain plan, sequence, and process information through repetition of interactive exercises. The individual performs thirteen different hand and foot exercises while auditory guide tones direct him or her to match the metronome beat. The difference between the individual's response and the computer-generated beat is measured in milliseconds (ms), and a score is provided. A low ms score indicates improved timing and overall performance. The program consists of either twelve or fifteen one-hour sessions that can be completed in three to five weeks.

The IM program has been shown to produce significant results in children and adults with a wide range of physical and cognitive difficulties, including ADD. The March–April 2001 issue of the *American Journal of Occupational Therapy* identified five core areas of statistically significant improvements gained through the IM program:

Attention and focus
Motor control and coordination
Language processing
Reading and math fluency
Ability to regulate aggression/impulsivity

IM also seems to improve golf scores. A study published in the *Journal of General Psychology* concluded that IM training improves golf accuracy as well as other complex motor activities. This program is worth looking into to help balance coordination and cognitive processing. You can learn more about it at www.interactivemetronome.com.

Brain Gym is a technique known worldwide to enhance learning and coordination. It was first developed by Dr. Paul Dennison in the early 1970s and involves a series of exercises designed to boost overall brain function. It has been reported to help both children and adults with ADD and learning disabilities and also helps to alleviate stress. In the 1970s it was already established that certain development movements were necessary for brain function. The theory is that activities, such as crawling, that stimulate both sides of the brain facilitate speech and language. But Dr. Dennison discovered that cross-crawl activities (touching the left hand to the right knee alternating touching the right hand to the left knee) worked by stimulating both the expressive and the receptive hemispheres of the brain and facilitated integrated learning. When you find yourself exasperated by your crawling child, you can relax in the knowledge that it is not only natural but a necessary stage in development. Many of my patients have reported benefits from Brain Gym

exercises. You can learn more about this technique at www.braingym
.com. Below are several examples of the exercises. Try a few to see if they
work for you.

BRAIN BUTTONS

How to do it: Make a C shape with the thumb and index finger of one
hand, and place them at either side of your breastbone just below the collar-
bone. Gently rub for 20 or 30 seconds while placing your other hand over
your navel. Then change hands and repeat. This reportedly helps with clear
thinking, "keeping place" while reading, crossing the visual midline for reading, and increasing energy for the task at hand.

LAZY-8S

How to do it: Extend one arm in front of your face. With your thumb
pointing upward, slowly and smoothly trace a large figure 8 on its side in the
air. Keep your neck relaxed and your head upright, moving only slightly as
you focus on the thumb and follow it around. This reportedly helps with
reading, speed reading, writing, and hand-eye coordination.

THINKING CAPS

How to do it: With your thumb and index finger, gently pull and unroll
the outer part of your ear, starting from the top and slowly moving to the
lobe. Pull the lobe gently. Repeat the whole exercise three times. This reportedly helps with spelling, self-awareness, short-term memory, listening ability, and abstract thinking skills.

CROSS CRAWL

How to do it: While standing, alternately touch your left knee with your
right hand, then your right knee with your left hand. Continue for 10 to 15
repetitions. This reportedly helps with reading, writing, listening, memory,
and coordination. It activates both sides of the brain simultaneously.

CALF PUMPS

How to do it: Stand an arm's length away from a wall, and place your hands
(a shoulder width apart) against it. Extend your left leg straight out behind
you so that the ball of your foot is on the floor and your heel is off the floor.
Your body is slanted at 45 degrees. Exhale, leaning forward against the wall
while also bending your right knee and pressing your left heel against the

floor. The more you bend the front knee, the more lengthening you will feel in the back of your left calf. Inhale, and raise yourself back up while relaxing and raising the left heel. Do the movement three or more times, completing a breath with each cycle. Then switch to the other leg and repeat. This reportedly helps with concentration, attention, comprehension, imagination, and the ability to finish tasks. This exercise removes the sense of being held back and not being able to join in.

Work to enhance your cerebellum through coordination exercises. Not only will it help you think more clearly and faster, it will help improve your judgment, attention, and overall brain health.

15

BRAIN SEX

MAKING LOVE IS GOOD FOR YOUR BRAIN

John turns his head toward a beautiful woman standing at the curb while sitting in his car at a long traffic light. His eyes instinctively go to her hair, her eyes, her lips, her breasts, her hips, and her shape. Her beauty is hypnotic. The vision is instinctively pleasurable, but it also holds him hostage. As the light turns, his eyes are glued to her as she crosses the street in front of his car; he watches how she moves, how her hair flows around her shoulders, and how her breasts gently bounce. As she passes him and walks away, he watches the movement of her bottom as she goes to the other side of the street. The moment is automatic, reflexive, and more powerful than any feeling on earth. Even when he tries to pull his attention away, an internal force drives him back to take another look. He is grateful that his wife isn't with him. It is so hard to keep his eyes from wandering when he is with her, even though he knows that she feels demeaned when he looks at other women in front of her. The male brain: very different from the female brain. The male brain is often driven by beauty, shape, fantasy, and obsession. It can leave a man quivering with pleasure, hoping for more, or it can hijack and ruin his life. The female brain is driven more often by language, communication, and bonding.

Even though it feels genital, sex occurs mostly in the brain. Your brain decides who is attractive, how to get a date, how well you do on the date, what to do with the feelings that develop, and how long those feelings last. Your brain is involved with everything you do, including everything sexual. It is the largest sex organ in the body (weighing about three pounds).

In the last three chapters we have focused on mental exercise, physical exercise, and coordination. Sex uses all three of these skills: mental exercise to socially connect with someone attractive; physical and coordination exercises to make the connection happen. As we will see, sex is a key to keeping the brain healthy.

This chapter will explore some brain basics about sexuality, such as how the brain becomes male and female and its role in attraction, attachment, commitment, and sexual performance, and then give you some practical tips to enhance the brain as it relates to your sexuality. Did you know that sexual competence and frequency have been associated with longevity? *Understanding the neuroscience of sexuality may save your life.* In a 1997 study published in the *British Medical Journal,* researchers from Queens University in Belfast tracked a thousand middle-aged men for over ten years and found that those who reported the highest frequency of orgasm enjoyed a death rate half that of those who lagged behind. In another study, men who had sex at least three times a week decreased their risk of a heart attack or stroke by half! Other studies have shown that regular sex improves sleep, moods, and testosterone levels. Research from the University of Pennsylvania reported that individuals who have sex at least once or twice a week show 30 percent higher levels of an antibody called immunoglobulin A, which is known to boost the immune system. Other studies have shown that frequent sexual activity is tied to lower risk of breast cancer in women and prostate cancer in men.

A word of caution: it is not indiscriminate sex that is associated with longevity. Random sex is associated with sexually transmitted diseases, such as syphilis and AIDS, both of which can shorten your life and destroy brain function. The sex described in this chapter is sexual activity with a committed, loving partner.

HORMONES AND THE BRAIN

HOW THE BRAIN BECOMES MALE OR FEMALE

The moment of conception determines whether you'll be male or female. Males get an X chromosome from their mothers and a Y chromosome from their fathers (XY), while females get X chromosomes from both their moms and their dads (XX). Inheriting a Y chromosome triggers two bursts of hormones, mostly testosterone, that change a male's brain and body. The first burst, early in the womb, produces a brain that is different from that of girls. From early in infancy, girl brains are more interested in smiles, communication, people, and security; boy brains are more interested in objects, actions, and competition. With higher levels of testosterone, the left parietal lobe, responsible for direction sense, visualizing objects in three dimensions (good for catching a football or watching a woman walk across the street), and mathematics becomes more highly developed. Without testosterone, the language centers of the brain become more developed, which is why girls like to talk and boys like to play catch. In addition, testosterone beefs up the area of the brain that is interested in sex. Not surprisingly, it is twice as large in men as in women.

The second burst of testosterone, during puberty, starts to turn a boy into a man. He now has twenty times the level of testosterone of most girls, his testicles descend, his voice deepens, his body becomes hairier, he has better-defined muscles, and he grows like a beanstalk. His mind becomes highly focused on girls; where before they were gross, now they are almost all he can think about. Bursts of estrogen and other female hormones help turn girls into women with breasts and rounder hips.

HOW LONG IS HIS RING FINGER?

According to University of Liverpool researcher John Manning, the size of a man's ring finger and genital are related to how much testosterone he received in the womb; the higher the testosterone level, the longer they are. In fact, looking at the length of a man's ring finger in comparison to his index finger will give an idea of the size of a man's penis. If the ring finger is longer, it means testosterone levels were healthy; if they are the same size or smaller, it means levels were lowered. Women can estimate the length of a man's penis by saying, "Show me your hands." Those who have unusually long ring fingers (indicating high testosterone) are also at greater risk for autism, dyslexia, stuttering, and immune dysfunction. A large member may not be all that great. On the other hand, a male with an unusually short ring finger is at higher risk for heart disease and infertility. Size matters, but it can go both ways.

BALANCED TESTOSTERONE FOR BRAIN HEALTH

Testosterone increases assertiveness and sexual interest. For some men, testosterone levels stay high throughout life; for others, they start to wane during middle age. Lower levels in teens tend to be associated with shy and unassertive behavior. In adult men, lower testosterone levels have been associated with low energy, decreased memory, poor work performance, decreased sexual desire and performance, and loss of strength and endurance. Low testosterone levels in females have been associated with decreased sexual interest. Small doses of testosterone are often prescribed to raise a woman's libido (not too much, however, as facial hair, aggression, and muscular biceps are generally not her goal).

ATTRACTION

WHY BEAUTIFUL WOMEN MAKE MEN STUPID

There is now scientific proof of something people have long suspected—beautiful women make men stupid. Canadian researchers showed men pictures of conventionally pretty and not-so-pretty women. The men rolled dice—and were told they could receive either $15 the following day or $75 after waiting a few days. The men who saw the pictures of the beautiful women were more likely to take the $15—proving, researchers say, that men stop thinking about long-term consequences once love chemicals kick in. (By the way, the same test was done on women—and men's attractiveness had no affect on their thinking processes.) Beautiful women seem to cause a man's limbic system to fire up (emotional charge) while his prefrontal cortex heads south, leaving the judgment area of the brain vacant. Las Vegas knows this principle very well. Casinos have beautiful waitresses dressed in low-cut, short dresses serving free alcohol—both lower PFC activity. No wonder the house has the edge.

HOW SHE LOOKS HIJACKS HIS BRAIN

When men get together, they often talk about how a woman looks and how she moves. Why? Thirty percent of the human brain is dedicated to vision. When a man sees an attractive woman, the visual areas of his brain fire with activity. She literally hijacks a large portion of his brain. It can feel emotionally overwhelming, even addictive. Using sophisticated imaging equipment, researchers from Emory University in Atlanta found that the amygdala, an area of the brain that controls emotions and motivation, was much more activated in men than in women when viewing sexual material for thirty minutes, even though both sexes reported similar levels of interest in the images. This may be one of the reasons men are much more interested in pornography than women. It is also no mistake that women spend more time caring for their physical appearance. How they look has much more impact on a man's brain than the other way around.

SPARKING ATTRACTION

When someone is attracted to someone else, areas deep in the brain, rich in the neurotransmitter dopamine, light up with pleasure. Dopamine neurons are involved with feelings of reward and motivation. This is the same area of the brain where cocaine works to produce a sense of euphoria. In addition, the brainstem gets into the act of attraction when sexy visual cues trigger the release of the adrenalinelike chemical phenylethylamine (PEA), the same chemical found in chocolate, which speeds up the flow of information between nerve cells. Taken together, the release of dopamine and PEA explains why, when we are around someone we are attracted to, we feel a "rush" and our heart beats faster. Attraction is a powerful drug.

IS BEAUTY ONLY SKIN DEEP?

Forget the idea that beauty is only skin deep. It is perceived in the brain, especially in the left front side. In a Spanish study, 160 different styles of artwork and 160 photos were presented to eight women. The brain's activity was recorded, and the results showed striking differences in the left side of the prefrontal cortex when they considered what was beautiful. The left PFC is also the happy side of the brain. When it is stimulated, people feel joy; when it is hurt, it often leads to depression and irritability.

Other researchers have suggested that men and women are attracted to symmetrical, fertile, healthy, younger-looking people. Your brain looks at a man or woman to decide whether you want your children to carry his or her genes. We look for signs of health, such as clear skin and bright eyes. The theory behind body symmetry is that asymmetrical features (such as eyes or breasts) suggest the presence of underlying health problems, thus yielding more troubled offspring. One of my patients was dating a woman with a lazy eye that diverted when she was tired. Even though he said he loved her, the asymmetry of her eyes bothered him, and he had no idea why.

NOSING AROUND WITH SEX

Smells trigger arousal and sexual response. Research shows that baby powder does it for women, cinnamon for men. There is a direct connection between your sense of smell in the olfactory bulb at the top of the nose and the erection center of the brain, called the septal nucleus. When cells in your olfactory bulb are stimulated in a certain way, it sends signals to the erection center to stand up and pay attention. Your brain gets an erection and sends signals lower in the body. Unpleasant smells, such as that of a man or woman who has not bathed recently, send a different set of signals that cause the septal area and the penis or clitoris to flatten. Researchers have found that people who have smell and taste disorders have a high frequency of sexual dysfunction. Measuring penile blood flow with what looks like a small blood pressure cuff, researchers found that sexual arousal in men was enhanced by the smells of lavender and pumpkin pie. Doughnuts, licorice, and cinnamon were also at the top of the list. No wonder Cinnabon is everywhere. In a women's study, increased vaginal blood flow, a sign of sexual arousal, was associated not with men's colognes (don't waste your money) but rather with baby powder. Women associate baby powder with freshly diapered, cute babies, and then they want one. A similar study found that women's sexual desire increased when they stood close to a nursing mother—close enough to smell her. Breastfeeding women and their infants produce a "chemosignal" that actually increases sexual desire in other women, according to research from the University of Chicago. While a chemosignal may not be perceived as an odor, it has a definite impact on mood and menstrual cycles when it's absorbed through the nose. "This is the first report in humans of a natural social chemosignal that increases sexual motivation," said lead researcher Martha McClintock in a news release announcing the study findings.

COMMITMENT

HIGHS AND LOWS OF NEW LOVE

When you meet someone who literally causes sparks to fly in your brain, hopefully the attraction is mutual. You find a special person and start spending more and more time with him. Attachment then starts to change your brain's chemistry. Several recent studies have shown that new love not only raises dopamine and PEAs (giving you a "high" sensation) but also starts to lower the neurotransmitter serotonin. Serotonin is involved with mood regulation and emotional flexibility. Low serotonin levels have been associated with obsessive-compulsive disorder, impulsivity, and excessive activity in the brain's anterior cingulate gyrus. When the ACG works too hard, people tend to get stuck on certain thoughts or behaviors (sounds like falling in love). Remember the last time you fell in love? All you could think about was your new love, and no matter how busy you were, you could always find time for her. Your moods were up when you thought about her, then went down when she didn't answer her cell phone the first time you called. You felt more reckless, and your friends wondered about your judgment. Lowered levels of serotonin make you vulnerable to depression if the relationship ends prematurely. In extreme cases, lowered levels of serotonin can trigger obsessive behavior, such as calling all the time, jealousy, or even stalking if your affection is not returned.

Several years ago one of my friends was scanned as part of our healthy study. Several months later he fell madly in love. One day he dropped by my office to tell me about his new love. I could hear in his voice that he was very taken with his new woman. I did a repeat scan on him just to see his brain in love. The second scan showed significant increased activity in the ACG, indicating that his brain was literally obsessed with this woman.

TO BE TOGETHER OR NOT TO BE TOGETHER

Oxytocin is an important hormone produced in the brain that is involved with bonding and attachment. When we feel connected, empathic, in love, the brain's emotional centers secrete higher levels of oxytocin. Women have naturally higher levels of this chemical, which boosts nonsexual bonding between a mother and newborn and is produced when a mother breastfeeds her baby. Usually low in males, orgasm causes oxytocin levels to skyrocket five times, making it easier for men to feel emotionally connected, keeping marriages alive. Dads with more of it stick around to help raise the kids. Oxytocin can be stimulated by touch, while making love or simply holding hands.

Love changes the brain. Oxytocin and serotonin are not as exciting to the brain as the dopamine and PEA released during the attraction stage, but they have longer effects and are part of the chemistry of what keeps us in love. After a while attraction chemicals cannot be sustained at such high levels. You start to notice your new love's asymmetries, and the intense feelings of euphoria and obsession start to wane. When you go through withdrawal from these chemicals, you begin to feel unbalanced and may even miss the high. You deal with the lowered pleasure chemicals either by becoming committed, because you truly love this new person and see real potential for the relationship, or by looking elsewhere for a new high.

WHY IS COMMITMENT EASIER FOR WOMEN?

Once you find an attractive partner, how does your brain decide if you want to keep him or her? Commitment is usually harder for men than women. Even though our goals are the same—continuity of the species—women are more oriented toward raising children. There is not one human society where men are primary caretakers for kids. Our brains are different. It doesn't mean that men don't help or that they are not essential in childrearing. We just have different roles. Unless women have experienced emotional trauma, they are usually more ready to settle down and start a family. This may frighten a man as he thinks about the responsibilities involved in raising children and being faithful to one woman, although this is easier for men with lower testosterone levels. An American study of more than four thousand men found that husbands with high testosterone levels were 43 percent more likely to get divorced and 38 percent more likely to have extramarital affairs than men with lower levels. They were also 50 percent less likely to get married at all. Men with the least amounts of testosterone were more likely to get married and stay married, maybe because low testosterone levels make men calmer, less aggressive, less intense, and more cooperative.

In addition to testosterone, another clue about commitment comes from new research on the hormone vasopressin. This chemical is involved in regulating sexual persistence, assertiveness, dominance, and territorial markings. Not surprisingly, it is found in higher levels in the male brain. Why do some men constantly live with the discomfort of a wandering eye, while others remain content with fidelity? The difference may have to do not only with testosterone but with this hormone as well. In male voles (little rodents), the levels of vasopressin seem to make the difference between stay-at-home dads and one-night-stand artists. The voles with a certain brain distribution of vasopressin were monogamous, while others with a different pattern were not.

Several other brain factors are important to the issue of commitment. People who have healthy activity in the prefrontal cortex can focus for longer periods of time, have greater empathy, and tend to make better husbands and wives. They are less prone to seek excitement, less impulsive, and more cooperative. People who have low activity in this part of the brain tend to be impulsive (more vulnerable to affairs), be easily distracted (trouble listening), get bored easily, and be on a constant search for the high that comes with new love. Low PFC activity is often associated with people who have ADD or who have had a brain injury. People who have too much activity in the PFC tend to be obsessive, oppositional, and argumentative. This behavior can push potential mates away. A healthy brain makes it easier to have a lasting, committed relationship.

ORGASM

CAN YOUR BRAIN HAVE AN ORGASM?

It seems as though you can't watch an hour of TV without seeing a commercial for Viagra, Cialis, or Levitra. Humans are definitely interested in enhancing sexual performance. From a brain science point of view, you can enhance your sexuality by stimulating the right hemisphere of the brain. As discussed, the brain is divided into two halves or hemispheres. The left side is more involved with language, logic, details, and planning, while the right side is more associated with music, rhythm, creativity, social skills, and spirituality. A number of studies have found that the right hemisphere, along with the limbic system, is involved with sexual pleasure and orgasm. Fascinating research has shown that people with right-hemisphere seizures can experience orgasm as a precursor to the seizure. In medical literature there are twenty-two reported cases of right-hemisphere seizures associated with the feeling of having an orgasm. In a study from Finland, eight male volunteers were studied with brain scans while they were having orgasm (must have been a fun study). The results showed overall decreased blood flow during orgasm in all brain areas except in the right prefrontal cortex, where the cerebral blood flow increased significantly.

WHY SHE CRIES OUT "OH GOD!" WHEN SHE'S HAVING AN ORGASM

The right hemisphere has also been talked about as the God area of the brain. When scientists stimulate the right hemisphere, people have more religious or spiritual experiences. They also report feeling the presence of God in the room. When she moans "Oh God, oh God," she may be connecting sexual pleasure to a deeper spiritual place in her brain. Music and dancing, which are often precursors to sex, enhance the right hemisphere.

WHY ORGASMS ARE BETTER THAN PAXIL

Orgasms can also have an antidepressant effect. They cause intense increased activity in the deep emotional parts of the brain, which then settle down after sex. Antidepressants tend to calm activity in the same part of the brain. People who engage in regular sexual activity experience less depression, and orgasm frequency may be one reason why. In addition, prostaglandin, a hormone found only in semen, is absorbed by the vagina and may have a role in modulating female hormones and moods.

OTHER BRAIN-SEX ISSUES

WHEN THINGS GET WEIRD

Weird sexual fetishes or fantasies ultimately are brain symptoms. They fall into the category of impulsive-compulsive disorders: impulsive because the person cannot control the behavior, and compulsive because even though he may want to stop, he cannot. A person who suffers from an obsession with voyeurism, exhibitionism, bestiality, S&M, or infantilism (being treated like a baby) often has too much activity in the emotional parts of the brain (as do people who have obsessive-compulsive disorders) and too little activity in the PFC or judgment center. A Harvard study of twenty-six men bothered by unusual sexual fantasies found that using medications to balance these two areas of the brain gave these men significant relief.

AFFECTION IS KEY TO HEALTH AND LONGEVITY

Regular sexual contact with a committed partner helps to keep your body and brain healthy. Don't avoid it with excuses about being too tired or too busy for physical affection. Also, try to avoid spending too much time at work to the exclusion of social endeavors. A lack of relationships sets us up to be depressed or to seek pleasure through solitary sexual activities, which are not as good for the brain. Men and women need touching, eye contact, and sexual connection to stay healthy. When you feel loved, nurtured, cared for, supported, and intimate, you are much more likely to be happier and healthier. You have a much lower risk of getting sick and, if you do, a much greater chance of surviving the illness.

AEROBIC SEX

One of the most compelling benefits of sex comes from studies of aerobic fitness. It is estimated that the act of intercourse burns about 200 calories, the equivalent of running vigorously for 30 minutes. Most couples average about 24 minutes for lovemaking. During orgasm, both heart rate and blood pressure typically double, all under the influence of oxytocin. A study conducted in Wales in the 1980s showed that men who had sex twice a week or more often experienced half as many heart attacks after ten years as men who had intercourse less than once a month.

MAKE SURE YOUR BRAIN WORKS RIGHT

Treat brain problems, such as depression or ADD, early so they don't interfere with your relationships and lovemaking opportunities. Some antidepressants, especially selective serotonin reuptake inhibitors such as Prozac and Lexapro, interfere with sexual function. Others, such as Wellbutrin, do not. Make sure to talk to your doctor if a medication is causing a problem.

WHY COFFEE AND CIGARETTES ARE THE ENEMIES OF SEX

Stay away from too much nicotine and caffeine. Both substances constrict blood flow to vital organs such as your brain and genitals. Less blood flow usually means less function.

WHY SHE BUYS SO MANY PAIRS OF SHOES

Women need sweet words, gentle touches, thoughtfulness, and especially foot rubs to get in the mood for sex. The foot sensation area of the brain is next door to the clitoral and penile areas, which may be one of the reasons that some women collect shoes and that some men have foot fetishes.

Erotic love is essential to human health. There is clear evidence that an active sex life leads to a longer life, better heart health, and better brain function.

Making love with a committed partner helps our bodies and brains work better.

MORE MONEY DOES NOT MEAN MORE SEX, BUT MORE SEX CAN MAKE YOUR BRAIN HAPPIER

There is positive news for people who have more activity in the bedroom than in their bank accounts. After evaluating the levels of sexual activity and happiness in sixteen thousand people, Dartmouth College economist David Blachflower and Andrew Oswald of the University of Warwick in England found that sex so positively influenced happiness that they estimated increasing intercourse from once a month to once a week is equivalent to the happiness generated by getting an additional $50,000 in income for the average American. In addition, they reported that despite what most people think, people who make more money do not necessarily have more sex. There was no difference, in their study, in sexual frequency among various income levels. The happiest people in the study were married people, who had on average 30 percent more sex than single folks. The economists estimated that a lasting marriage equated to the happiness generated by an extra $100,000 annually, while divorce depleted an estimated $66,000 annually worth of happiness. Taking care of your marriage can save you lots of money.

SUMMARY OF SOME OF THE HEALTH BENEFITS OF REGULAR SEXUAL CONTACT

For women, in research studies, regular sex with a partner has been associated with:
- More regular menstrual cycles
- More fertile menstrual cycles
- Lighter periods
- Better moods
- Better memories
- Increased pain relief
- Better bladder control
- Fewer colds and flu
- Reduced stress

- Staying in shape
- Increased youth-promoting hormone DHEA
- Increased testosterone and estrogen
- Weight control—sex burns about 200 calories per half-hour, yoga 114, dancing (rock) 129, walking (at 3 mph) 153, weight training 153

For men, regular sex with a partner has been associated with:

- Increased heart rate variability (a sign of heart health and a calmer mind)
- Improved heart cardiovascular function (three times a week decreased the risk of heart attack or stroke by half)
- Higher testosterone levels (stronger bones and muscles)
- Improved prostate function
- Improved sleep

16

IMPROVING REALITY

THE BRAIN'S ROLE IN PERCEPTION

The mind is its own place, and in itself
Can make a heaven of hell, a hell of heaven.

John Milton, *Paradise Lost* (1667)

Your brain creates your reality. It is not what happens to you in life that determines how you feel; it is how your brain perceives reality that makes it so. Most people are unaware that they are controlled not by events or people but by the perceptions their brain makes of them. I once heard the following story: at the turn of the last century, a shoe company sent a representative to Africa. He wired back, "I'm coming home. No one wears shoes here." Another company sent its representative, and he sold thousands of shoes. He wired back to his company, "Business is fantastic. No one has ever heard of shoes here." Their brains perceived the same situation from different perspectives, and they obtained opposite results. The view that your brain takes of a situation has more reality in it than the actual situation itself. Noted psychiatrist Richard Gardner once wrote that the world is like a Rorschach test, where a person is asked to describe what he or she sees in ten inkblots that mean absolutely nothing. What we see in the inkblots and what we see in life is based on our inner view of the world formed in neural connections.

PERCEPTION AND REALITY

Our perceptions bear witness to our state of mind and the state of our brain. A calm limbic or emotional brain leads to more rational thought; an overactive limbic brain is associated with greater anxiety and sadness. An enhanced left hemisphere is associated with happy or optimistic perceptions; while an overactive right hemisphere (or low left hemisphere) is associated with fear and negative thinking. As our brain functions, so do we perceive. Therefore, in reality, we should seek to change not only the outside world but our own brains and attitudes. It is how your brain perceives situations, rather than the actual situations themselves, that causes you to react. I often write this equation for my patients:

$$A + B = C$$

A is the actual event,
B is how we interpret or perceive the event, and
C is how we react to the event.

Most people think the A things in life, what happens to us, determine our behavior. In large part, it is actually the B stuff. Other people or events (A) cannot make us do anything. It is our brain's interpretation or perception (B) that causes our behavior (C). Here are two examples.

STEPHANIE

Stephanie overheard a discussion at lunch between her husband and her stepdaughter about a trip they were all planning the following summer. Stephanie heard only part of the conversation and thought they were planning the itinerary without her input. She became irate and stormed out of the restaurant. As Stephanie replayed the event for me during a marital therapy session—sure she had interpreted the whole event correctly even though her husband said she was mistaken—I wrote on a pad of paper, A + B = C. The conversation between her husband and stepdaughter was A; her interpretation was B; and her storming out of the restaurant was C. I asked Stephanie if she could have reacted in any other way. At first she said no, she knew what she saw. But then logic helped to soften her position. Reluctantly, she said other intentions were possible, and perhaps she misinterpreted what happened—the B stuff. She had actually never tried to give input on the trip but just fumed when she was not specifically asked her opinion. She was sensitive to her stepparent role and had trouble being assertive in asking for what she wanted.

IAN

Ian, twenty-four, came to our clinic in Newport Beach from Minnesota for problems with drug abuse and ADD. He was having family troubles and was taking much longer than expected to get through college. His brain SPECT study showed marked decreased activity in the prefrontal cortex (consistent with ADD) and scalloping throughout the surface of his brain (consistent with the drug abuse). When he saw his scan (the event, A stuff) he became visibly upset, thought he was brain damaged and hopeless (his interpretation, B stuff), and stormed out of my office (his reaction, C stuff). He came back a few minutes later wanting to hear the rest of the explanation about his scan. Before we talked more I wrote out the equation $A + B = C$. We talked about his interpretation (B stuff) and how it had caused him to overreact (C stuff). In fact, his scan was very good news. He already knew that he was having problems, because that was why he came more than two thousand miles to see me. The scan showed damage from drugs, but if he stopped, the damage was likely to heal over time. If he kept using the drugs, it would worsen. That piece of information was critical, so he could make better decisions and stop using drugs. The evidence of ADD on his scan was also very important because doctors had suspected ADD through the years but were never sure. Now we were sure of his diagnosis and could get him the proper help. Good news. When he listened and understood what his scan really showed, he was more relaxed and had hope that things could be better (new B stuff and a new attitude).

Just as the brain can distort reality, it can also improve it. So much begins in the brain. Balancing your brain through diet, exercise, music, stress reduction, and supplements will help your perceptions. At the same time, balancing and improving your perceptions can help balance the brain. Psychotherapy— or therapy for your thoughts, feelings, and behaviors—has been found to actually enhance brain function. How your brain works is certainly involved in how you think, feel, and act, but how you think, feel, and act can also influence brain function. The brain and behavior help or hurt each other.

Researchers in the last decade have shown that many different forms of psychotherapy help to balance brain function. Several studies have shown that cognitive therapy (teaching people to correct negative thought patterns and to think in more rational, positive ways) enhances brain function. A Canadian study found that cognitive therapy helped not only to heal depression but also to balance brain function in a similar way to medication (but without the side effects or expense of medication). Other research groups from Canada and Sweden came to the same conclusions. The Swedish study took eighteen patients with significant social anxiety and divided them into three groups: one received an antidepressant, one received cognitive therapy, and a third did not receive any treatment. Both the antidepressant and the cognitive therapy groups improved (also showing improvement on brain scans), while the group that did not get help stayed the same. One of my favorite studies comes from Canada, where researchers examined twelve patients who had paralyzing spider phobias. They performed imaging studies while the patients looked at pictures of spiders and showed that during that time one of the brain's fear centers exploded with activity. Then these patients were taught cognitive therapy to deal with their fears of the tiny arachnoid creatures. After treatment they were rescanned while looking at the same spider pictures. This time the fear centers were calm. Therapy for thoughts helps change brain function. Change your thoughts, change your brain!

In the same way, changing your relationships can change your brain. A landmark study from UCLA found Interpersonal Psychotherapy (ITP), which teaches people to get along better with others by improving social support, communication, conflict resolution, and assertiveness training, to be an effective cure for depression. ITP also helps to reset brain function, enhancing prefrontal cortex activity (improving focus and judgment) and calming limbic activity (making one feel more positive).

A number of studies have found that patients with obsessive-compulsive disorder (repetitive bad thoughts or inappropriate behaviors) are helped by behavior therapy. Behavior therapy involves telling the brain that certain behaviors are not only irrational and but also symptoms of the brain working too hard and fooling the person. It teaches patients to change counterproductive behaviors, stop the bad thoughts that come into their minds, and wait out urges to do compulsive behaviors rather than just give in to them and expose them to their fears. Three different brain-imaging studies found that, like medication, behavior therapy can help bring healing to suffering patients and balance the brain. In this disorder the brain works too hard, especially in the basal ganglia (anxiety) and the anterior cingulate gyrus (gear shifter). Behavior therapy helps to settle down or rebalance these areas. Change your behavior, change your brain.

One of the most interesting scans that I have done through the years were those of a psychologist, Noelle Nelson, who was at the time writing a book titled *The Power of Appreciation* (now in print). She wanted to be scanned after spending a half-hour meditating on all the things she was thankful for in her life. In that scan her brain looked healthy. I then asked her to do one more scan after thinking about all the things she hated in her life. I felt that we needed a comparison scan to see the difference that an attitude of gratitude can make in the brain. Reluctantly, she agreed, even though she knew that thinking about the things she hated in life would make her feel bad. They did. She thought about her fears of getting sick, of being unable to work or to support her animals. She thought that if her dog got sick and died because she was out of work, she would get depressed and never recover. Her second scan was very different from the healthy gratitude scan: both her cerebellum and her left temporal lobe were deactivated (Images 16.1–16.4). Decreased cerebellar activity is associated with decreased motor coordination and thought coordination. People get clumsier and less able to think their way out of problems. Lowered left temporal lobe activity is associated with dark thoughts and memory problems. Negative thought patterns change the brain in a negative way. Being grateful for the wonderful things in your life literally helps you have a brain to be grateful for.

CHANGING YOUR REALITY

Here are five steps to improve your brain and your reality.

1. DO NOT BELIEVE EVERY FIRST THOUGHT YOU HAVE.

It is easy to misunderstand or misperceive a situation. Think about all of the brain systems involved in communication—sight and sound processing, decoding meaning, and comparing incoming information with past experiences. You can see how some things can get miscommunicated. Whenever you feel slighted, hurt, or negated by someone else, try to get a clarification of the situation. Clear communication can solve many relational problems. Feed your brain accurate information, not just gut feelings. Correct your perceptions, change your brain.

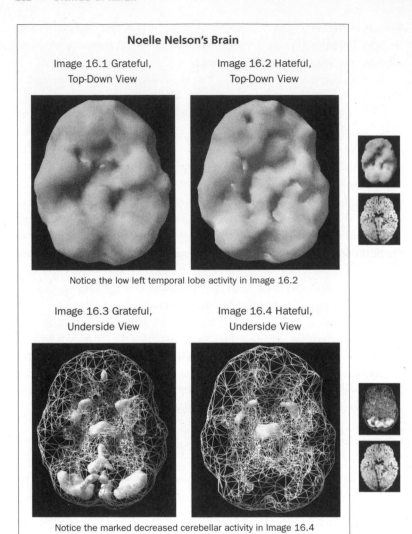

Noelle Nelson's Brain

Image 16.1 Grateful,
Top-Down View

Image 16.2 Hateful,
Top-Down View

Notice the low left temporal lobe activity in Image 16.2

Image 16.3 Grateful,
Underside View

Image 16.4 Hateful,
Underside View

Notice the marked decreased cerebellar activity in Image 16.4

2. REALIZE THAT YOUR THOUGHTS ARE EXTRAORDINARILY POWERFUL.

Every time you have a thought, your brain releases chemicals. Every time you have a positive, happy, hopeful, grateful thought, your brain releases chemicals that help you feel better and have more efficient brain function. Whenever you think awful, miserable, negative thoughts, your brain works less efficiently and is likely to put you into an emotional slump. Learn how to direct your thoughts to see the glass as half full. Your brain works better with positive thought fuel than with negative energy.

3. RECOGNIZE THAT THOUGHTS LIE, ARE EASILY DISTORTED, AND CAN ROB YOU OF JOY.

People who suffer from depression, anxiety, and panic disorders are filled with what I call ANTs, automatic negative thoughts. They tend to predict the worst and focus on whatever is negative about a situation. It is as though an ANT infestation is sucking the life force out of the physical brain. If you suffer from this problem, it is important to develop an internal anteater to rid yourself of these pests and their nests. Whenever you feel sad, mad, or nervous, write out what you are thinking. You will notice that many of those thoughts are irrational and hurtful. The act of writing down the ANTs takes away their power by turning off their emotional food supply and eventually choking the life out of them, allowing you to replace them with more helpful thoughts. Kill the ANTs, change your brain.

4. USE THE PLACEBO EFFECT.

Your brain takes what it sees and makes it happen. Negative thoughts can make negative things happen, while positive thoughts can help you reach your goals. The expectation of success is a very powerful force by itself. Skilled physicians have known for centuries that positive expectations play a crucial role in healing many illnesses. Until about 150 years ago, medical therapeutics mainly involved the doctor-patient relationship and the placebo effect. (A placebo is an inert substance that has no physiological effect on a problem.) Actually, most treatments by physicians in times past would have been more harmful than beneficial to patients, if it weren't for their faith in the healing powers of the treatments and their own recuperative powers. The benefits of the placebo effect are determined by the expectations and hopes shared by the patient and the doctor. According to Dr. T. Findley, action, ritual, faith, and enthusiasm are the vital ingredients. Dr. Jerome Frank, after studying the psychotherapeutic process, concluded that the therapist's belief in his treatment and the patient's belief in the therapist were the most important factors in effecting a positive outcome.

Although placebos are pharmacologically inert, they are by no means "nothing." They are potent therapeutic tools, on average about one-half to two-thirds as powerful as morphine in relieving severe pain. One-third of the general population are placebo responders in clinical situations relating to pain, whether the pain is from surgery, angina, cancer, or headache. Placebo responses are clearly not simply a result of patients fooling or tricking themselves out of pain—placebo administration can produce real physiological changes. Some of the physiological pathways through which placebo effects work have been identified. In 1978 a University of California research team found that the placebo effect of pain relief in dental patients could actually be blocked by administering naloxone, a drug that neutralizes the effects of morphine in the body. This study and others have made it clear that belief in pain relief stimulates the body to secrete its own pain-relieving substance. These endorphins act in the same manner as morphine. In one brain-imaging study, researchers found that when a placebo worked for depressed patients, their brain function also changed in a positive way. Change your beliefs, change your brain.

5. TELL YOUR BRAIN WHAT YOU WANT, AND MATCH YOUR BEHAVIOR TO GET IT.

Since your mind takes what it sees and makes it happen, it is critical to visualize what you want and then match your behavior over time to get it. Too many people are thrown around by the whims of the day, rather than using their prefrontal cortex to plan their lives and follow through on their goals.

THE ONE-PAGE MIRACLE

A powerful yet simple exercise that I have designed is called the One-Page Miracle, so named because it has quickly focused and changed many people's lives. It will help guide nearly all of your thoughts, words, and actions for brain health.

Take a sheet of paper, and clearly write down your major goals. Use the following three main headings: Relationships, Work/Finances, and Self. Under "Relationships," write the subheadings of Spouse/Lover, Children, Family, and Friends. Under "Work/Finances," write down your current and future work and financial goals. Under "Self," write down your goals for your physical health, emotional health, spirituality, and interests. Your self is the part of you that is outside your relationships and your work. Often it is the part of you that no one sees but you.

Next to each subheading succinctly write down what's important to you in that area. Write what you want, not what you don't want. Be positive, and use the first person. Write what you want with confidence and the expectation that you will make it happen, and include what you are currently doing to make it happen. Keep the paper with you so that you can work on it over several days. After you finish the initial draft (you'll frequently want to update it), place this piece of paper where you can see it every day, such as on your refrigerator, by your bedside, or on the bathroom mirror. In that way, every day you will focus your eyes on what's important to you. This makes it easier to match your behavior to what you want. Your life will become more conscious, and you will spend your energy on goals that are important to you.

I separate the areas of relationships, work, and self in order to encourage a more balanced approach to life. Burnout occurs when our lives become unbalanced and we overextend ourselves in one area while ignoring another. For example, in my practice I see that a common cause of divorce is that one person works so much that little energy is left over for his or her spouse.

EXAMPLE

John is a sixty-two-year-old married college professor who has three adult children and two grandchildren.

JOHN'S ONE-PAGE MIRACLE

What Do I Want? What Am I Doing to Make It Happen?

RELATIONSHIPS

Wife/Sandy	Enjoy time together, spend special time each week
	I treat her as special as she really is to me
	I'm improving our communication
	I support her in whatever she chooses to do for herself
Children:	I am involved in their lives, show love and support
	I encourage them and remember what it was like to be their ages
Grandchildren:	A special relationship of unconditional love and support
	Spend time with them each month doing some special activity

Friends:	I continue to spend time with special friends
	I nurture new friendships as I meet special people
Family:	I am involved with members of my family in a positive way
	I stay out of the politics of the moment and am less reactive to the buttons my younger sister pushes in me
WORK	I do my best work for my students
	I engage in activities that further help the university grow
	I continue my professional education and develop my professional interests
	I do charity work to give back to my profession
FINANCES	I will make a net income of approximately $200,000
	I save 15–20 percent of my net income to invest
	I am accumulating enough money to live where I want
	I am investing in a retirement fund monthly
SELF	
Emotional:	I am more even-tempered, I am not upset by little things
	I am more positive and optimistic
Physical:	I eat a diet that helps me feel better and live longer
	I walk thirty minutes a day and maintain my weight between 160 and 165
Interests:	I enjoy keeping up with current events
	I continue to enjoy working on restoring old radios
Spirituality:	I continue to search for meaning every day
	I go to church to have a group of people with whom to worship and pray

Let your brain help you design and implement your life goals. Work toward achieving goals that are important to you. Many other people or corporations are happy to decide what you should do with your life. Use the One-Page Miracle to help you be the one who has the say.

Your brain receives and creates reality. Give it some direction to help make your life what you want it to be.

MY ONE-PAGE MIRACLE

What Do I Want? What Am I Doing to Make It Happen?

RELATIONSHIPS

Spouse/Love: _____

_____

_____

Children: _____

_____

_____

Friends: _____

_____

Family: _____

_____

WORK _____

_____

FINANCES _____

_____

SELF

Brain: _____

_____

Physical: _____

_____

Interests: _____

_____

Spirituality: _____

_____

SERENADE THE BRAIN

MUSICAL INTERVENTIONS

If I had to live my life again I would have made a rule to read some po-
etry and listen to some music at least once a week; for perhaps the
parts of my brain now atrophied could thus have been kept active
through use.

—Charles Darwin, *Autobiography* (1887)

Simply put, music moves us.

At three o'clock one cold winter morning in the year 2000, I found myself crawling out of bed to take my teenage daughter and her friends to the Oakland Coliseum box office to stand in line to buy 'N Sync tickets. The night before Breanne had told me that she and a group of her friends were going to Oakland to try to get great seats for the concert. It was well known at my house that she was in teenage love with JC, one of the group's lead singers. I didn't even consider allowing her to go alone. But rather than disappoint her with my first impulse—"There is no way in hell you are going to Oakland at three A.M. with a group of your girlfriends"—I decided to go along. When we got to the parking lot, even in the dark we could see a very long line of teenage girls waiting anxiously to purchase tickets. As we got in line, the box office staff handed out lottery tickets. Breanne got the number four, which meant she was fourth in line, among hundreds. As we bought the tickets, I heard her squeal with joy as she got front row center seats. All the way to and from the Coliseum, Breanne and her friends sang 'N Sync songs. I had literally never seen her so happy. The night of the concert Breanne was enraptured by seeing her teen idol perform right in front of her. In fact, she said later that JC's sweat dropped on her as he performed and that she would never shower again. (Thankfully she gave up that idea.) She was so happy. I, of course, couldn't hear for a week. I sat up in the rafters with my younger daughter. The sound of fifteen thousand teenage girls screaming ruined any potential enjoyment from the concert. The pitch of female teenage voices still frightens me to this day.

Why does music move us? Why is it such an important part of our lives? Does the brain have a role in music? Can music be healing? Does it have any dangers, besides blasting out one's eardrums? This chapter will explore these questions and provide some suggestions for using music to help make a good brain great.

HOW THE BRAIN LISTENS

Babies come into the world wired for music. In the mother's womb, they respond to songs in the environment. At about four months old they begin to fuss when they hear music they do not like and coo along with melodies that please them. Music is in our genes. At an early age our musical capacity is shaped by the culture in which we live. Our background affects how our instruments are made, how we hear sounds when others sing, and even how we hear music. I have a Lebanese heritage but was born in the United States. Since I was never exposed to Arabic music at a young age, I often find it grating and uncomfortable. But friends and colleagues who were born in the Middle East love it. Through the brain, music interacts with our environment to create our likes and irritations. Certain types of music can enhance brain function, memory, and emotion, while other forms of music can cause us problems. Music is powerful.

As we have seen, the human brain is divided into two hemispheres. Typically, the right hemisphere has been identified as the seat of music, but there is not just one area in the brain responsible for music. In making and listening to music we use both sides; music is an interplay of many functions. It is exactly for this reason that music is healing and has the ability to enhance brain function. Music integrates the whole brain.

Some cerebral circuits respond to certain types of music; these circuits may also be involved in processing other forms of sound. The part of the brain that hears pitch is also involved in understanding speech. Sound enters the ears and goes to the auditory cortex in the temporal lobes. The right temporal lobe is important for hearing pitch, melody, harmony, and rhythm. The left side of the brain is usually better at hearing changes in frequency and intensity, both in music and in words. The left side analyzes incoming data. The right side helps to put music together into a whole piece. Novices tend to listen to music as a whole, with the right side, while musicians tend to hear music with the left hemisphere as they analyze the content of the musical form. The limbic brain processes the emotional aspects of music as well, triggering memories.

Music triggers emotions and emotions trigger memories. Hearing "our song" at a wedding anniversary can bring tears of joy and emotional connection; but hearing "our song" three years after a divorce can trigger tears of intense sadness and loss. Music has great power to move our emotions.

SING

It used to be easy to tell if I was in a good mood in the morning. I would start singing when I rolled out of bed. When I was sad, anxious, or irritated, I would be wrapped up in my own misery and little sound would come out. Once I recognized the pattern, I started to sing no matter how I felt. Singing has healing qualities (even if you are like me and are not very good at it). It expands the lungs and increases the flow of oxygen to the body and brain. It wakes us up and stimulates the rhythms of life. Singing and music (not always the same thing) have been connected to intelligence, creativity, emotion, and memory. When you put certain information to a tune, such as "The ABCs" (a Mozart piece), you are more likely to remember it. Singing stimulates temporal lobe function, an area of the brain heavily involved in memory. When you can sing new information, put it to a tune, you are more likely to remember it.

Preschool and kindergarten teachers use singing to enhance learning. So why do we stop singing in the second or third grade? Perhaps we should continue the singing into later grades. When I was a basic trainee in the military, we often sang when we marched. I still have those songs in my head. When we sang as a group, morale and energy went up, and the tasks that we were doing didn't seem quite as bad (like twenty-mile road marches). Sing whenever and wherever you can. You may have to sing softly if your voice is like mine, so as not to irritate others. Sing loudly if your voice is beautiful. In a similar way, humming can also make a positive difference in mood and memory. Mozart hummed as he composed. Children hum when they are happy. Adults often hum tunes that go through their minds, lifting their spirits and tuning their mind. Consciously focus on humming during the day. As the sound activates your brain, you will feel more alive and your brain will feel more tuned in to the moment.

MUSIC, MEDITATION, AND SPIRITUAL EXPERIENCE

With the sponsorship of the Alzheimer's Prevention Foundation, my colleagues and I teamed up with Dr. Dharma Singh Khalsa and Dr. Nisha Money to study the impact of meditation on the brain. We chose a simple twelve-minute form of meditation, Kritan Kriya, that is easy for busy people to practice. It is based on five primal sounds: saa, taa, naa, maa, and aa. Meditators chant each sound as they consecutively touch their thumb to fingers two, three, four, and five. The sounds and fingering are repeated for two minutes out loud, two minutes whispering, four minutes silently, two minutes whispering, and two minutes out loud. We performed SPECT scans on the participants when they were at rest one day, and then after meditation the next day. We saw marked decreases in the left parietal lobes (which showed a decreasing awareness of time and space) and significant increases in the prefrontal cortex (which showed that meditation helped to tune people in, not out). We also observed increased activity in the right temporal lobe, an area that has been associated with spirituality. Our meditators found that finding amusing. "Of course," one said, "that is why we meditate."

The fact that music enhances spiritual experience should come as no surprise—nearly all major religions have music as part of the worship service. Brain science gives us some clues as to why. Music is processed in the right temporal lobe, the same area that is now referred to as the God spot in the brain. Neuroscience researchers have found that stimulating the outside of the right temporal lobe also stimulates religious and spiritual experience. In addition, insight (or the "aha" experience) also activates the right temporal lobe. Music has the potential to stimulate both spiritual experience and insight. When you are faced with a difficult problem, it may be a good idea to play some music and allow your brain to work on the puzzle while it listens. Music helped Thomas Jefferson write the Declaration of Independence.

When he could not figure out the right wording for a certain part, he would play his violin. The music helped him get the words from his brain onto the paper.

LEARN A MUSICAL INSTRUMENT

If you always wanted to learn a musical instrument, now is the time. Learning to play a musical instrument enhances brain function. It teaches the brain new patterns and stimulates wide areas of the cortex. Music has the capacity to enhance how we think, reason, and create. The data is impressive. Experiments using Mozart's Sonata for Two Pianos in D Major (K448) produced short-term enhancement of the right hemisphere, which helps us see images in three-dimensional pictures (visual spatial reasoning). Additionally, preschool children who received piano keyboard lessons for six months improved their performance dramatically on a visual spatial reasoning task, with the effect lasting for days, whereas control groups (including a computer control group) did not improve. In a follow-up study by researchers at the University of California at Irvine, thirty-four preschoolers were given piano keyboard training. After six months all the children could play basic melodies from Mozart and Beethoven. They exhibited significant increases in visual spatial skill (up to 36 percent improvement) compared with other preschoolers who received computer lessons or other types of stimulation. The College Entrance Examination Board in 1996 reported that students with experience in musical performance scored 51 points higher on the verbal part of the SAT and 39 points higher on the math section than the national average. In a study of approximately 7,500 students at a university, music majors had the highest reading scores of any students on campus. Learning a musical instrument, at any age, can be helpful in developing and activating temporal lobe neurons. As the temporal lobes are activated in an effective way, they are more likely to have improved function overall.

Many other studies have highlighted the need to keep music an important part of our educational process. A study from the University of Sarasota and East Texas State University found that middle school and high school students who participated in instrumental music scored significantly higher in standardized tests than their nonband peers. University studies conducted in Georgia and Texas found significant correlations between the number of years of instrumental music instruction and academic achievement in math, science, and language arts. In another study, students who were exposed to a type of music-based lessons scored a full 100 percent higher on fractions tests than those who learned in the conventional manner. (These second- and third-grade students were taught fractions in an untraditional manner— using basic music rhythm notation: they were taught about eighth, quarter, half, and whole notes. Their peers received traditional fraction instruction.) In a study that premedical students will find fascinating, music majors were the most likely group of college grads to be admitted to medical school. Lewis Thomas studied the undergraduate majors of medical school applicants. He found that 66 percent of music majors who applied to medical school were admitted—the highest percentage of any group. For comparison, 44 percent of biochemistry majors were admitted.

College-age musicians are emotionally healthier than their nonmusician counterparts. A study conducted at the University of Texas looked at 362 students who were in their first semester of college. They were given three tests, measuring performance anxiety, emotional concerns, and alcohol-related problems. In addition to having fewer battles with the bottle, researchers also noted that the college-aged music students seemed to have surer footing when facing tests. A ten-year study, tracking more than 25,000 students, shows that music-making improves test scores. Regardless of socioeconomic background, music-making students get higher marks in standardized tests than those who have no music involvement. The test scores studied were not only from standardized tests, such as the SAT, but also from reading proficiency exams.

The world's top academic countries place a high value on music education. Hungary, the Netherlands, and Japan stand atop worldwide science achievement and have a strong commitment to music education. All three countries have required music training at the elementary and middle school levels, both instrumental and vocal, for several decades. The centrality of music education to learning in the top-ranked countries seems to contradict the United States' focus on math, science, vocabulary, and technology.

MOVE WITH THE MUSIC

Music is sensory, emotional, and motor—we feel the music, and it literally moves us. Music is as much about action as it is about perception. When music engages our brain—when performers play or listeners tap, dance, or sing along—the experience of music is often coupled with action. Simple coupling might be foot-tapping to a beat, whereas more complex coupling would be dancing a waltz, singing a song, or playing a melody on a violin. Passionate coupling may be making love to music, such as Ravel's *Bolero*.

One example of the healing power of music comes from George I of England. King George had problems with memory loss and stress management. He read from the Bible the story of King Saul, recognized that Saul had experienced the same type of problems that he was experiencing, and realized that Saul overcame his problems by using special music. With this story in mind, King George asked George Frederick Handel to write some special music for him that would help him with his memory loss and stress in the same way that music helped Saul. Handel wrote his *Water Music* for this purpose.

MOZART FOR FOCUS

In one controlled study, Mozart has been found helpful for ADD children. Rosalie Rebollo Pratt and colleagues studied nineteen children, ages seven to seventeen, with ADD while playing recordings of Mozart during three-times-a-week brain-wave biofeedback sessions. *One Hundred Masterpieces*, volume three, *Wolfgang Amadeus Mozart* was the music used. It included the selections from Piano Concerto no. 21 in C, Flute Concerto no. 2 in D, *The Marriage of Figaro, Don Giovanni,* and other concertos, sonatas, and operas. The group that listened to Mozart reduced their theta brain-wave activity (slow brain waves are often excessive in ADD) in exact rhythm to the underlying beat of the music, and they displayed better focus and mood control, diminished impulsivity, and improved social skill. Among the subjects that improved, 70 percent maintained that improvement six months after the end of the study without further biofeedback training.

CAN MUSIC HELP IN HEALING?

Understanding the neuroscience of music will allow us to harness its healing power. Studies have shown that following heart bypass surgery, patients in intensive care units where background music is played needed lower doses of drugs than patients in units where no music is played. Some hospitals play soft background music in intensive care units for premature babies. Such music, as well as a nurse's or mother's humming, helps the premature babies gain weight faster and leave the unit earlier than those who don't hear these sounds. At the other end of life, music has been used to calm Alzheimer's patients. Mealtime in nursing homes can be a struggle, but certain types of music have been shown to reduce confusion and irritability. In a University of Louisville Medical School study of retired nuns in two nursing homes, researchers introduced the playing of recorders and other instruments as the only change in the environment. They discovered significant improvements in memory; playing music, reading notes, and moving fingers all worked to enhance memory.

Researchers have also found that music lowers blood pressure in certain situations and increases oxygen consumption by the heart. Researchers in Rome used music therapy as an additional treatment for severely brain-injured patients. The therapy consisted of musical improvisation between the patient and therapist by singing or by playing different musical instruments, according to their own unique abilities. Thirty-four patients were studied who had been in a coma for an average of fifty-two days. The results of the study showed that patients who had music therapy had a significant reduction of undesired behaviors such as inertia or agitation.

THE MUSIC YOU LISTEN TO MATTERS!

After she heard me lecture on music and the brain, my 'N Sync daughter, Breanne, did a study with twelve of her friends for a psychology class. She timed them playing the game Memory while they listened to nothing, Mozart, rock, heavy metal, and rap music. She found that they did best at the game when they listened to Mozart (even better than those listening to nothing at all), and worst when they listened to heavy metal and rap music.

Below are some suggestions of music that I find personally healing.

Don Campbell, *Mozart as Healer: Classical Healing for the New Millennium*

Don Campbell, *Essence: The Ambient Music of Don Campbell*

———, *Healing Powers of Tone and Chant*

Michael Hoppé, *Solace*

David Lanz, *Beloved*

Andrew Weil, *Self-Healing with Sound and Music*

Ralph Vaughan Williams, et al., *Inner Peace for Busy People: Music to Relax and Renew*

The following wonderful titles by Dean Evenson are available at www. soundings.com:

Arctic Refuge
Ascension to Tibet
Healing Dreams
Healing Sanctuary
Music for the Healing Arts
Native Healing
Peace Through Music

OTHER FORMS OF ART

Even though this chapter has focused on music, other forms of art (visual art, photography, poetry, and prose) are also helpful for developing and enhancing brain function. Since the brain makes art, encouraging its study and appreciation must be useful to enhance brain function.

SOOTHING THE BRAIN

CALMING THE STRESS THAT KILLS CELLS

Most people think of stress as bad. Actually, stress is both good and bad. Stress is good because it causes us to pay attention to what is going on around us: in traffic, with our finances, at work, and in our relationships. Stress can motivate us (to study for an exam or pay our bills on time); it can protect us (we buy alarm systems for our homes, businesses, or cars); and it can feed us (we go to work to put food on the table). When something is stressful to us, it usually means that we should be paying attention to it.

But stress is bad when it overloads our resources. Too much stress can actually kill you. Chronic stress has been implicated in anxiety and depressive disorders, obesity, Alzheimer's disease, heart disease, and a host of immune disorders, including cancer. When stress hits, levels of adrenaline (leading to anxiety) and cortisol (leading to many ills discussed below) increase, while levels of the hormones DHEA and testosterone (leading to loss of muscle tissue, increased fat, and decreased libido) decrease. Both adrenaline and cortisol are released by the adrenal glands (located above the kidneys) in response to real or perceived stress. The human brain is so advanced that even imagining a stressful event will cause the body to react to the perceived threat as if it were actually happening. We can literally scare our body into a stress response. The brain is a powerful organ.

Adrenaline and cortisol help us deal with acute stress by increasing energy when we face a threat. They are the primary chemicals of the fight-or-flight response. Whenever you confront an immediate perceived threat, such as a rattlesnake in your front yard (which happened to me not too long ago), the body prepares either to run away or to fight the threat. The hypothalamus, located in the deep emotional brain, releases a chemical called CRF (corticotropin-releasing factor), which in turn stimulates the pituitary gland to produce ACTH (adrenocorticotropin hormone), which in turn stimulates the adrenal glands to produce cortisol and adrenaline. Together these chemicals prepare the body to fight or flee. Among other things, adrenaline dilates our pupils (increasing visual acuity); shunts blood from our hands and gut to the large muscles of arms and legs (so we can fight or run); increases our breathing rate and heart rate (to increase oxygen to the body); and increases sweat gland activity (to keep us cool). Cortisol stimulates the release of glucose, fats, and amino acids into the bloodstream for energy production.

The problem with stress in our modern world is not these short bursts of adrenaline and cortisol—we need those reactions to deal with our rattlesnake encounters. The problem is that for many of us the stress reaction never stops—traffic, bills, bosses, employees, unhappy in-laws, too little sleep, illnesses, and too much to do. Chronic exposure to adrenaline causes our systems to be overstimulated and leads to anxiety and depression, obesity, and memory problems. Chronic exposure to cortisol can make us fat and stupid.

In normal amounts, both of these chemicals are essential. Cortisol, for example, has an initial anti-inflammatory effect. (Doctors use cortisol-like medications to help with asthma, arthritis, and colitis and to relieve certain skin disorders.) It also calms immune response in organ transplantations. In appropriate amounts, both chemicals help the body maintain internal balance. Low levels of cortisol are associated with Addison's disease, an illness where stress can cause a dangerous drop in blood pressure and even circulatory collapse. President John F. Kennedy had Addison's disease and had to take cortisol tablets when he was under great periods of stress, such as during the Cuban missile crisis. High levels of cortisol are related to an illness called Cushing's disease, where people have an accumulation of central body fat (making them look pear-shaped) and muscle wasting of the limbs (skinny arms and legs). Cushing's disease can be associated with immune system problems, psychotic depression, and many other health issues.

Cortisol levels can be elevated by chronic stress, intense exercise, pregnancy, depression, anxiety, and the intake of stimulants such as ephedra and caffeine (as little as two or three cups a day). When Marine recruits are exposed to high levels of stress (such as extreme sleep deprivation or intellectual or physical stress), they have increased cortisol blood levels and decreased performance. Extreme-endurance athletes have increased cortisol levels as well as decreased testosterone levels, leading to reduced sperm counts and reduced libido. Excess in any form is stressful.

Chronic exposure to high levels of cortisol has been associated with myriad problems that make us unhappy, such as increased appetite, sugar and fat cravings, and abdominal obesity. Cortisol signals fat cells to hold on to their fat stores, leading to a high waist-to-hip ratio (WHR), in which your waist size is large compared to your hip size, making you look like a pear. A person's WHR is associated with perceived attractiveness. An optimal WHR is 0.8; anything above that puts a person at risk for illnesses (mentioned above) associated with higher cortisol levels. A WHR ratio of 0.7 has been associated with the most attractive women, in part because it is a sign of health and potential fertility. As we age, our figure goes from being an hourglass to being a shot glass (especially if we are drinking too much alcohol or eating too much sugar).

Long-term exposure to high levels of cortisol has also been associated with low energy, poor concentration, elevated cholesterol levels, heart disease and hypertension, increased risk for strokes, diabetes (reduced sensitivity to insulin), muscle wasting, osteoporosis, anxiety, depression, irregular menstrual periods, lowered libido, and decreased fertility. High cortisol levels decrease immune system function, shrinking the thymus gland and impairing white blood cell function (by as much as 50 percent following a severe stress). Chronic stress dramatically increases the use of medical services and raises health care costs. Stress not only increases cortisol, it decreases key anabolic hormones such as DHEA, growth hormone, and testosterone. This combination causes you to store fat, lose muscle, slow your metabolic rate, and increase your appetite.

In the last decade we have become aware of a clear association between chronic stress, high cortisol levels, and memory problems, causing shrinkage of cells in the hippocampus of the brain. In fact, people with Alzheimer's disease have higher cortisol levels than normal aging people.

SOOTHING THE BRAIN

Okay, it makes sense that too much stress is bad for the brain. So what can you do? Get even more stressed out from worrying about it? No, but it all starts with accepting that stress is a problem and with using your prefrontal cortex to do something about it. Unfortunately many people have to experience an emotional threat to life itself before they start taking their health seriously: a heart attack, cancer, stroke, or a bout with depression. Once we have been limbically challenged, our resources kick into gear and we start exercising and changing our lives. Hopefully you won't need that jolt, but if you do, think about your family surviving without you. Having grown up Roman Catholic, I am never above using guilt—in fact, reasonable guilt can help keep one's behavior in check. Your behavior provides a model for your children. If you are living a healthy, balanced life, your children are more likely to follow in your steps. If you are living an extreme, out-of-control, stressed-out life, you are teaching them to do the same thing. Okay, now that we have guilt in the mix, let's get down to destressing your life. Here's an eleven-step plan.

1. Recognize that too much stress can make you sick and hurt your brain. The research is clear and compelling. No one can completely avoid stress, but it is critical to take stress seriously.

2. It is okay to say no and to renegotiate your commitments. Being too busy leaves no time for stress-reducing activities. Too often we agree to do things without first asking ourselves if the request fits into our own lives. Many people say yes without first processing the request through their prefrontal cortex. When someone asks you to do something, a good first response might be, "Let me think about it." Then process the request through your time, desires, and goals. In a typical week I get asked to do many, many things, more than I could possibly do. Saying no used to stress me out. I did not want to disappoint anyone. I somehow had the thought that I should be able to do everything people asked of me. Then one day, as I looked at an impossible mountain of work, I finally just said no. I asked myself whether I really wanted to do these things, if they fit the goals I had for my life, and if they were good for me. If they did not meet my criteria, I started to say no. It was hard at first, until I realized I was saving my own life. If you are doing too much, do the important things (which has to include taking care of your health and your brain) and renegotiate the rest.

3. Get enough sleep. Getting less than six and a half hours of sleep at night decreases our ability to fight stress. Research has shown that people who consistently get less sleep than others have overall decreased brain function. Inadequate sleep may promote insulin resistance: compared with those who sleep seven and a half to eight hours at night, those who get fewer than six and a half hours secrete 50 percent more insulin and are 40 percent less sensitive to insulin. Lowered sleep has been associated with diabetes and obesity. In our fast-paced society, we are often sleep deprived. In 1910 adults got an average of nine hours of sleep each night; in 1975 it had decreased to seven and a half; and in 2000 it has decreased further, to seven hours. Here are some tips to get better sleep if you struggle with insomnia.

- Eliminate watching television one or two hours before bedtime, especially any program that may be overstimulating or anxiety provoking, such as the news.

- Some people are successful reading themselves to sleep, but read boring books. If you read action-packed thrillers or horror stories, you are not likely to drift off into peaceful never-never land. Sometimes I read the Book of Numbers in the Old Testament or a biochemistry textbook.

- A warm, quiet bath before bed is often helpful.

- A bedtime backrub may be soothing. Starting from the neck and working down in slow rhythmic strokes can be very relaxing. Some children and teens say that a foot massage is particularly helpful (although it may be hard to find someone to give a teen a foot massage if they haven't showered or taken a bath before bed).

- Soft, slow music often helps people drift off to sleep. Instrumental music, as opposed to vocal, seems to be the most helpful.

- Nature-sounds tapes (rain, thunder, ocean, rivers) can be very helpful. Others like the sound of fans.

- A mixture of warm milk, a tablespoon of vanilla extract (not imitation vanilla, the real stuff), and a tablespoon of sugar can be very helpful. It will increase serotonin to your brain and help you sleep.

- Meditate or do self-hypnosis (see pages 172–173)

- Use sleep control therapy. Many sleep experts give these tips to chronic insomniacs to help them get to sleep on a regular basis.
    - Go to bed only when sleepy.
    - Use the bed and bedroom only for sleep.
    - When you are unable to fall asleep or return to sleep easily, get out of bed and go into another room, and return to bed only when sleepy.
    - Maintain a regular rise time in the morning regardless of sleep duration the previous night.
    - Avoid daytime naps.

• Sometimes medications are needed if getting to sleep is a chronic problem. There are pros and cons to using medication sleep aids. On the positive side, medications tend to work quickly and can help normalize a disturbed sleep pattern. On the negative side, they can have side effects (such as grogginess in the morning) and you can become dependent on them if you take them for too long. It is best to think of medications for sleeping problems as a short-term solution. Use the other ideas first.

4. Regular exercise is one of the best stress-busters on the planet. See Chapter 14.

5. Use regular prayer and/or meditation. Maintaining a regular prayer life or meditative practice creates many health benefits, mostly by calming the stress response. Physicians Larry Dossey (*Healing Words*), Dale Matthews (*The Faith Factor*), and others have written books outlining the scientific evidence for the medical benefits of prayer and other meditative states. Some of these benefits are: reduced feelings of stress, lower cholesterol levels, improved sleep, reduced anxiety and depression, fewer headaches, more relaxed muscles, and longer life span. People who pray or read the Bible every day are 40 percent less likely to suffer from hypertension than others. A 1998 Duke University study of 577 men and women hospitalized for physical illness showed that the more patients used positive spiritual coping strategies (seeking spiritual support from friends and religious leaders, having faith in God, praying), the lower their level of depressive symptoms and the higher their quality of life. A 1996 survey of 269 family physicians found that 99 percent believed prayer, meditation, and other spiritual and religious practices can be helpful in medical treatment; more than half said they currently incorporate relaxation or meditation techniques into the treatment of patients.

Using brain SPECT imaging, Andrew Newberg and his colleagues at the University of Pennsylvania investigated the neurobiology of meditation, in part because it is a spiritual state easily duplicated in the laboratory. They scanned nine Buddhist monks both before and during prolonged meditation. The scan revealed distinctive changes in brain activity as the mind went into a meditative state. Specifically, activity decreased in the parts of the brain involved in generating a sense of three-dimensional orientation in space. Losing one's sense of physical place could account for the spiritual feeling of transcendence, being beyond space and time. They also found increased activity in the prefrontal cortex, which is associated with attention span and thoughtfulness. Meditation seemed to tune people in, not out. A functional brain-imaging study of transcendental meditation (TM) showed calming in the anterior cingulate gyrus and basal ganglia, diminishing anxiety and worries and fostering relaxation.

6. Practice self-hypnosis to calm the brain. Like meditation, self-hypnosis is a powerful tool to help balance brain function and decrease stress. I became fascinated with hypnosis during medical school and took a one-month elective in it my senior year. It was a pivotal decision in my life because it taught me to appreciate other forms of self-healing. Hypnosis and meditation have similar effects on the body. Imaging studies have found that hypnosis helps balance brain function. Studies from Belgium and Canada have shown that hypnosis increases the attention areas of the brain and the left hemisphere; it also decreases the perception of pain and the areas of the brain that perceive pain. Self-hypnosis can be a powerful tool for many different reasons, including help with sleep. When I was a medical intern at the Walter Reed Army Medical Center in Washington, D.C., many patients asked me for sleeping pills to help with the insomnia that goes with being sick in a noisy hospital. Before I gave them pills, I would hypnotize them and make them a self-hypnosis tape. Eight times out of ten they no longer needed the sleeping pills.

Here are instructions on how to put yourself into a simple hypnotic trance. Do not try to do this while driving or operating heavy machinery.

- Focus your eyes on a spot, and count slowly to twenty. Let your eyes feel heavy as you count, and close them as you get to twenty.
- Take three or four very slow, deep breaths.
- Tighten the muscles in your arms and legs, then let them relax.
- Imagine yourself walking down a staircase while you count backward from ten. (This will give you the feeling of "going down" or becoming sleepy.)
- With all of your senses (sight, touch, hearing, taste, smell) imagine yourself in a very sleepy scene, such as lying by a fire in a mountain cabin or in a sleeping bag at the beach.
- After spending ten to fifteen minutes in your special place, allow yourself to come back to full consciousness. If you fall asleep, it means that likely you are not getting enough sleep.

Try it. I still use this technique when I am stressed.

7. **Become your own biofeedback machine.** Biofeedback uses instruments to measure physiological processes in the body that are related to stress and teaches people how to self-induce calming states. Biofeedback teaches people to warm their hands, relax their muscles, dry their skin, slow and deepen breathing patterns, calm excessive brain-wave activity, and increase heart rate variability. All of these responses counteract the fight-or-flight response. As I mentioned, under stress our bodies produce more adrenaline, which triggers the fight-or-flight response. Our hands become cold, to shunt blood to the large muscles of the arms and legs so we can fight or run; our hands sweat to cool off our bodies; our breathing becomes fast and shallow; our heart beats faster and is less variable to try to meet our body's increased demand for oxygen; our muscles tighten to get us ready to fight or run; and our brain waves heighten to increase our alertness. Learning how to self-regulate these functions through mental exercises gives us a sense of being in control, which improves our ability to deal with stress. There are many biofeedback therapists across the United States. A wonderful website to learn more about biofeedback and to find practitioners in your area is www.aapb.org.

It is beyond the scope of this book to tell you how to do biofeedback, but I want to tell you about a very cool biofeedback video game you (and your kids) can do at home. I am generally opposed to video games because I do not think they help the brain develop properly. But this particular game is very cool. It is the ultimate video game in that you play it exclusively with your mind. It is called Experience the Journey into the Wild Divine (www.wilddivine.com). It is not very expensive (about $160) and comes with everything you need, including sensors to measure hand sweat-gland activity and heart rate variability. The graphics of the game beautifully instruct players how to relax their minds and get into a healthful physiological state. When your body goes into the relaxed state, you can blow pinwheels with your mind, juggle balls in the air with your brain power, and fly a balloon.

8. **Avoid substances that stress the brain.** It should be obvious, but many people are not aware that excessive amounts of caffeine and nicotine can cause damage to the brain. These substances both constrict blood flow to the brain and can cause premature aging. In addition, substances that people use as uppers—such as ephedra, synephrine, yohimbine, and guarana—cause increased brain stress.

9. Consider stress-busting supplements. Some supplements may be helpful in counteracting stress. B vitamins are especially effective. During heightened periods of stress people may also benefit from St. John's wort, 5-HTP, SAMe, L-theanine, or valerian. Take these under the supervision of your health care professional. Just because something is natural does not mean it is completely innocuous.

10. See a psychotherapist. If you are chronically stressed, it may be a good idea to see a psychotherapist to talk about your problems and learn better skills in dealing with stress. Many people have a negative attitude about psychotherapists, but I think of them as life consultants. When a great business has troubles, it is likely to deal with the problems head-on and find the best consultants to help. We should behave the same way in our personal lives. In dealing with stress I often refer people to biofeedback therapists, hypnotherapists, and therapists in EMDR (see Chapter 8), which helps them deal with anxiety, past traumas, and performance enhancement.

11. Get more laughter into your life. A growing body of scientific literature suggests that laughter counteracts stress and is good for the immune system. According to University of California at Irvine's Lee Berk, "If we took what we know about the medical benefits of laughter and bottled it up, it would require FDA approval." Laughter can lower blood pressure, trigger a flood of endorphins (the brain chemicals that can bring on euphoria and decrease pain), and enhance our immune systems. Gamma-interferon, a disease-fighting protein, rises with laughter. So do B-cells, which produce disease-destroying antibodies, and T-cells, which orchestrate the body's immune response. Laughter lowers the flow of dangerous stress hormones that suppress the immune system, raise blood pressure, and increase the number of platelets, which cause clots and potentially fatal coronary artery blockages. The average child laughs hundreds of times a day. The average adult laughs only a dozen times a day. If only we could collect those lost laughs and use them to our advantage.

One person was able to do this quite effectively. In Norman Cousins's classic book *Anatomy of an Illness,* he describes how he used laughter to treat a debilitating immune disorder called ankylosing spondylitis. The illness cause him pain, fatigue, and a great deal of anxiety. He believed that he became sick because he was overtired from travel and work and his body was in a state of adrenal exhaustion. He went from doctor to doctor, took medicine after medicine, and was not getting better. One specialist estimated his chances of recovery at one in five hundred. In partnership with his physician, he gradually stopped taking all of his medications, added large doses of intravenous vitamin C, and began a program of laughter. Allen Funt, famed producer of the television series *Candid Camera,* sent him films of the TV series, along with a projector for his laughter therapy. Cousins also watched Marx Brothers and Laurel and Hardy films. He discovered that ten minutes of a genuine belly laugh had a pain-relieving effect and would give him restful sleep for two hours. He laughed and laughed. After a period of time his illness started to improve, and eventually it went away.

Put laughter in your life every day. Watch comedies (a helpful form of TV), go to comedy clubs, read joke books (my favorite is *The Far Side* by Gary Larson, which is pretty sick, but I am a psychiatrist after all), and swap jokes with your friends. Abraham Lincoln suffered from serious periods of depression. He used laughter and telling jokes as one form of medicine. Here are three of my favorite humorous Lincoln sayings.

- Common-looking people are the best in the world: that is the reason the Lord makes so many of them.
- If I were two-faced, would I be wearing this one?
- It is said that an Eastern monarch once charged his wise men to invent him a sentence to be ever in view, and that should be true and appropriate in all times and situations. They presented him with the words: "And this, too, shall pass away."

KEEPING THE BRAIN YOUNG

PREVENTING PROBLEMS OF AGING

The lights in the brain dim with age, unless we actively work to keep it healthy. The Amen Clinics' database of more than thirty thousand scans of people from three to one hundred years old make it clear that the normal brain has fewer and fewer resources with age (see Table 19.1). There is less blood flow to bring oxygen and glucose to the neurons and take away waste products, and there are fewer antioxidants to protect it against free radical formation and to lower hormone levels to keep it young. This is the fate of the typical brain. But your brain does not have to succumb to age at the same rate as others. There are simple things you can do today to prevent disease and keep your brain healthy for as long as possible. This chapter will teach you how to recognize and reduce your risk for the diseases of aging that affect the brain.

In order to stay healthy, the brain has to repair itself on a constant basis. It's not like a car that you can take into a garage for a tune-up or to have a part replaced. Your brain has mechanisms to repair damage as a result of the normal wear and tear of life. The hardware of the brain—neurons, dendrites, axons, synapses, and others—must be cared for. The brain has to maintain its hundred billion neurons if they are to consistently function well. If the number of neurons in any cortical circuit decreases by more than one-third—as is the case in Alzheimer's disease—the circuit can no longer compensate for the loss, and symptoms appear.

Many people still believe that we are born with all of the nerve cells we will ever have and that human brains simply cannot replace dead neurons. Scientists once considered brain damage irreversible and neurological disease in

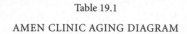

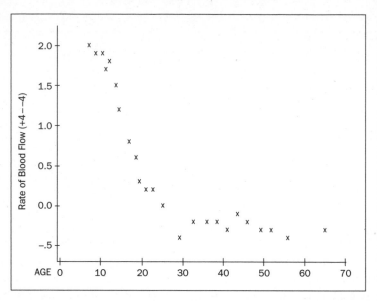

Over time the brain becomes less and less active (unless we do things to keep it healthy and balanced). This chart, based on our research on more than four thousand people, shows what happens to the cerebral cortex over time. The numbers on the vertical axis represent the scaled readings of the brain scans; they are plotted against age, from 0 to 70. As you can see, adolescence is a time of tremendous change—no wonder we struggle as teens. Brain activity stabilizes until about 45, then starts to dip once again. Using the strategies in this book, you can help keep your brain healthy with age.

the elderly unstoppable. In stunning new research, however, investigators demonstrated that adult human brains generate new cells after all. Since then scientists have been furiously studying the implications, and research in this area has accelerated.

Neurogenesis means "birth," but this birth cycle is begun by death. Let's say you go to a New Year's Eve party and have a little too much champagne. You come home and sleep it off. By the time you awaken, several hundred thousand neurons have died from alcohol toxicity. Somehow the number of neurons in your brain has to be brought back up to normal to reach a steady state. Neurogenesis is the process that develops and maintains the functional capacity of the circuits by replacing neurons that are killed or damaged. The very act of the neurons dying triggers certain growth factors in the brain to stimulate the formation of new neurons.

Neurogenesis doesn't know when to stop; left on its own it will continue creating new neurons until the brain explodes. The brain has to regulate itself so that just the right numbers of neurons are maintained. When the number generated reaches a certain level, cell death is triggered, which miraculously brings the number back down. Yet once again this death mechanism does not know when to stop killing, and thus new neuron formation is triggered again. This process allows the brain cell growth to stay within a certain range, so that the circuits can always function well—at least under normal conditions.

This brain repair process is called synaptic plasticity, neurogenesis, and cell death. You can think of it simply as the brain's governor, whose main job is to govern the population. It must maintain the right homeostasis, or all hell will break loose. Not only do the numbers of cells have to be regulated, but so do the one thousand trillion synapses that connect them. Maintaining synaptic health is essential for brain function.

Diseases of aging in the brain typically cause the following problems:

- They reduce the number of brain cells, as in Alzheimer's disease.
- They reduce the number of connections between cells, which happens when there is depression or a lack of mental or physical exercise.
- They impair the generation of electrical activity, which can happen if one consumes three or more alcoholic drinks at a time.
- They disrupt cell machinery to produce energy, which happens in Parkinson's disease and diabetes, and in chemotherapy and radiation therapy for cancer.
- They damage axons to slow the speed of signals in the brain, as in hypertension, heart disease, stroke, and head trauma.

KNOW AND REDUCE YOUR RISK FOR THE DISEASES OF BRAIN AGING

The following list contains the risk factors for diseases of brain aging. The number in parentheses indicates how significant the risk factor is. For example,

2.0 means that there is twice the risk of having a problem; 4.0 means that the risk is quadrupled. Check the ones that apply to you.

1. _____ (3.5) One family member with Alzheimer's disease or other cause of dementia
2. _____ (7.5) More than one family member with Alzheimer's disease or other dementia
3. _____ (2.0) A single head injury with loss of consciousness for more than a few minutes
4. _____ (2.0) Several head injuries without loss of consciousness
5. _____ (4.4) Alcohol dependence or drug dependence in past or present
6. _____ (2.0) Major depression diagnosed by a physician in past or present
7. _____ (10) Stroke
8. _____ (2.5) Heart (coronary artery) disease or heart attack (myocardial infarction or MI)
9. _____ (2.1) High cholesterol (hyperlipidemia)
10. _____ (2.3) High blood pressure (hypertension)
11. _____ (3.4) Diabetes
12. _____ (3.0) History of cancer or cancer treatment
13. _____ (1.5) Seizures in past or present
14. _____ (2.0) Limited exercise (less than twice a week or less than thirty minutes per session)
15. _____ (2.0) Less than a high school education
16. _____ (2.0) Jobs that do not require periodically learning new information
17. _____ (2.3) Smoking cigarettes for ten years or longer
18. _____ (2.5) One apolipoprotein E4 gene (if known)
19. _____ (5.0) Two apolipoprotein E4 genes (if known)

_____ **Total Score** (Add up the numbers in parentheses for all items checked.)

INTERPRETATION

If your score is 0, 1, or 2, then you have low risk factors for developing the brain diseases of aging.

If your score is 3, 4, 5, or 6, then you have a moderate risk for developing the diseases of aging and should take prevention seriously.

If your score is greater than 6, then prevention strategies should be part of your everyday life.

GENETIC RISK FACTORS

A family history that includes memory problems is a cause for concern and preventive action. This is especially true for people who have a first-degree relative (mother, father, brother, or sister) with Alzheimer's disease, strokes, or Parkinson's disease. Several genes are associated with Alzheimer's disease and other causes of memory problems, especially the E4 version of the apolipoprotein E (apoE) gene on chromosome 19. Everyone has two apoE genes, and if one of them—or worse, two of them—are apoE4, that person's chances of getting memory problems is quite high. Of course, apoE genes alone are not dangerous; we need them to function, but the E4 type increases our risk of age-related problems. There are three versions of the apoE gene: E2, E3, and E4, and it is the last one that is the culprit. As with all genes, we inherit one copy from each parent, and any one person could have the following combination:

E2/E2, E2/E3, E2/E4,
E3/E3, E3/E4, or
E/4, E/4.

If a person has two E4 genes, it means he received one from each parent. For about 15 percent of the general population, at least one of the two apoE genes is the E4 gene. People who have no apoE4 gene at all have only a 5 to 10 percent chance of developing Alzheimer's disease after age sixty-five, whereas people with one apoE4 gene have about a 25 percent chance. Given the increased risk of problems with this gene, it would be wise to know your apoE genotype. To find out what it is, you can ask your doctor to order a simple blood test. As I've mentioned, this should be done under the strictest confidence so that insurance companies or others cannot obtain the information and potentially use it against you. It would be best to pay for the test on your own and keep it in your personal records; do not allow it to be included in your medical records.

ALCOHOL AND DRUG ABUSE

Alcohol is a double-edged sword. It can increase the risk of stroke, heart disease, and possibly Alzheimer's. Five percent of all strokes in the United States are alcohol-related. Four or more drinks a day increase the risks for stroke and heart disease, while one drink every few days actually reduces these risks (presumably by increasing HDL cholesterol, which clears other types of cholesterol that cause hardening of the arteries).

Clearly, drug abuse damages the brain. More than a hundred brain imaging studies demonstrate that drug abuse—including cocaine, methamphetamines, marijuana, heroin, and other opiates—diminishes brain function and damages neurons. One of the first things I learned from doing brain imaging on a wide variety of psychiatric patients was that drug abuse damages the function seen on SPECT scans. I have made several posters that hang in more than twenty thousand schools, prisons, and drug abuse treatment centers nationwide on the effects of drugs on brain function. Recently, it was found that cocaine inhibits a part of cells involved in energy production, which has also been linked to Parkinson's disease.

Reducing the risk of aging from alcohol and drug abuse is simple—stop using the things that harm brain function. If drinking is a problem, I recommend stopping altogether and seeking treatment if needed. If it is not a problem, limit yourself to no more than one or two normal-size drinks a week.

CANCER AND CANCER TREATMENT

In addition to cancers that invade the brain and can cause dementia, some treatments for cancer get into the brain and can also cause dementia. But there are few studies on this issue. One of the studies done examined the effect of chemotherapy in a hundred women with breast cancer. Dr. E. S. van Dam found that women who received chemotherapy plus tamoxifen were four to eight times more likely to develop cognitive impairment than early-stage breast cancer women who had not received chemotherapy. A review of children who are long-term survivors of cancer, particularly brain cancer and leukemia, showed that the two most common long-term effects of radiation therapy and chemotherapy are cognitive and hormonal impairment. Surprisingly, they found that the cognitive impairment is progressive and not static. Anything you do to decrease the risk of cancer—such as exercise, eating more fruits and vegetables, decreasing stress, and stopping smoking—will also help your brain stay healthy.

CARDIOVASCULAR DISEASE

All forms of cardiovascular disease increase brain aging. The heart and blood-vessel system delivers blood and nutrients to the brain. Whatever is good for the heart is good for the brain; whatever is bad for the heart and blood-vessel system is bad for the brain. Forms of cardiovascular disease include atherosclerosis, coronary artery disease, congestive heart disease, heart rhythm problems, high cholesterol, and hypertension.

The most effective way to prevent cardiovascular problems is to prevent the diseases that produce them. Exercise and diet are both important factors that you have some control over. You can also investigate your family history. If it includes heart disease, stroke, diabetes, or high cholesterol, then you should consult your physician and ask her to screen for these conditions at the appropriate age of risk or after the age of forty in general. An annual screening after the age of fifty is extremely wise. Regular cardiovascular exercise for thirty minutes or more goes a long way to improve lipid metabolism to reduce lipid deposits in blood vessel walls. The main focus of your diet should be to reduce saturated fats, which are high in the bad cholesterols and contribute to the fatty deposits in the blood vessels that cause atherosclerosis. Foods high in saturated fats include butter, cheese, cookies, doughnuts, pastries, ice cream, fatty meat, and so on. (See Chapter 11 for more information on a brain-healthy diet.)

CEREBRAL VASCULAR DISEASE (BRAIN BLOOD-VESSEL DISEASE)

The risk of developing serious brain problems in a person who has a stroke is six to ten times greater than in the general population. Even a stroke smaller than a pencil-head eraser increases the risk for dementia four- to twelvefold.

A stroke is a single damaging attack, but the risk factors that lead to a stroke, such as high blood pressure, smoking, heart disease, and diabetes, develop over a long time. You can reduce your stroke risk by taking the following simple steps:

- Keep blood pressure under control. Check your blood pressure often, and if it is high, follow your doctor's advice on how to lower it. Treating high blood pressure reduces the risk for both stroke and heart disease.
- Stop smoking. Cigarette smoking is linked to increased risk for stroke and heart disease. The risk of stroke for people who have quit smoking for two to five years is lower than for people who still smoke.

- Exercise regularly. Exercise makes the heart stronger and improves circulation. It also helps control weight. Being overweight increases the chance of high blood pressure, atherosclerosis, heart disease, and adult-onset (type 2) diabetes. Physical activities like walking, bicycling, swimming, and tennis lower the risk of both stroke and heart disease. Talk with your doctor before starting a vigorous exercise program.
- Eat a healthy, balanced diet and control diabetes. If untreated, diabetes can damage the blood vessels throughout the body and lead to atherosclerosis.

The warning signs for stroke are: sudden numbness or weakness in the face, arm, or leg, especially on one side of the body; sudden confusion, trouble speaking or understanding; sudden trouble seeing in one or both eyes; sudden trouble walking, dizziness, loss of balance or coordination; sudden severe headache with no known cause. If you suspect that either you or someone you know is having a stroke, call 911 immediately, even if the symptoms seem to have gone away. Sometimes the warning signs last for only a few minutes and then disappear, but that does not mean the problem is resolved. You could have had a transient stroke, called a transient ischemic attack (TIA), and although it doesn't last long, it is a symptom of a greater medical problem. Don't ignore a TIA—see your doctor right away.

DEPRESSION

Depression has been associated with increased risk for dementia. A prior history of medically treated depression can be associated with a threefold increase in this risk. In an impressive study, Drs. Kristine Yaffe and Terri Blackwell from the University of California at San Francisco studied the association between depression and cognitive decline. As part of an ongoing prospective study, they evaluated 5,781 elderly women. They studied them at baseline and again four years later, using tests for depression, memory, and concentration. At baseline, 211 (3.6 percent) of the women had six or more depressive symptoms. Only 16 (7.6 percent) of these women were receiving treatment, which meant 93.4 percent of depressed woman in the study were not being treated. Increasing symptoms of depression were associated with worse performance at baseline and follow-up on all tests. Women with three to five symptoms of depression were at 1.6 greater odds for cognitive deterioration, while women with six or more symptoms of depression were at 2.3

greater odds for problems, more than double the risk. They concluded that depression in older women is associated with both poor cognitive function and subsequent cognitive decline. It is critical to note that most psychiatric diseases in general are, in effect, brain diseases. Schizophrenia, for example, has been shown to affect the frontal and temporal lobes, and depression has been associated with decreased activity in the frontal lobes. These illnesses are also exacerbated by chronic stress; increased stress hormones have been shown to kill cells in the hippocampus.

Early treatment is essential to stave off the ravages of psychiatric illnesses. Our work with SPECT teaches us that with appropriate treatment, the brain becomes more balanced and works in a much more efficient way. Treatment can involve medication, psychotherapy, supplements, or a combination of all three. Medication and supplements work by altering certain neurotransmitters in the brain—for example, antidepressants, which work by enhancing serotonin, norepinephrine, or dopamine. Psychotherapy has also been shown recently to affect neurotransmitter systems and enhance activity seen on SPECT and PET scans.

DIABETES

Diabetes damages almost every organ, including the brain, by making blood vessels hard and brittle. This increases the likelihood of stroke, heart disease, and hypertension, all of which increase aging problems for the brain. In diabetes there is a failure to keep blood sugar (glucose) at appropriate levels, which impairs memory and other cognitive functions. Sometimes the treatment of diabetes lowers blood glucose too much (hypoglycemia), which can also impair memory and other cognitive functions.

People with a family history of diabetes should have a fasting blood glucose test once a year after the age of forty. Also, if symptoms of increased urination, increased thirst, or increased appetite develop, then fasting blood glucose should be checked for diabetes. One of the most effective preventions against diabetes is exercise, which improves insulin's ability to regulate blood glucose. Although there are many reasons why daily exercise is better than exercise every three days, the available data suggest that exercising *at least* every three days helps protect against diabetes and a number of other illnesses. A diet high in refined sugars increases the risk of diabetes. A balanced diet, such as the one recommended in *The Zone,* is a good approach to eating that helps stabilize blood sugar. Consulting with a nutritionist or dietitian is also a good idea.

LACK OF EDUCATION

A number of studies that attempted to identify risk factors for dementia have noted an inverse relationship between education and dementia—the more education, the less dementia. This is a controversial risk factor because educational background and achievement can introduce a number of other factors that generally affect health and opportunity. Despite the controversy, significant evidence supports the idea that education (and increased mental activity) produces a functional reserve in the brain, which can provide protection against developing dementia. The philosophy of "use it or lose it" is very much at play in the brain. The more it is challenged and stimulated (without overdoing it—which leads to the harmful effects of stress), the more ability it will have as we age. No one that I am aware of has studied whether learning disabilities and other conditions, such as ADD, that often lead to school failure are associated with dementia. My strong suspicion is that there is a connection. Any condition that negatively impacts brain function can put the brain at risk for other problems later on. I believe we should aggressively treat children and teens with school problems so that they will stay in school and hopefully grow to love learning and be the lifelong learners they need to be to help protect their brains.

Keeping your mind active—by reading, doing crossword puzzles, traveling, taking classes, and otherwise acquiring knowledge outside your typical or usual experience—helps to reduce the risk of aging problems.

HIGH HOMOCYSTEINE LEVELS

Homocysteine is an amino acid regulated by folic acid in red blood cells. If levels are elevated, homocysteine increases risks for coronary artery disease, stroke, and dementia. The risk is largely eliminated for homocysteine levels of 10 or below. High homocysteine levels in the blood increase LDL cholesterol, which narrows the coronary blood vessels. A study of persons who required coronary angioplasty (to open up their coronary arteries) showed that homocysteine levels higher than 11 could be treated with folic acid (1 mg), vitamin B12 (400 mcg), and pyridoxine (10 mg) to reduce the level to about 7. This homocysteine reduction helped prevent renarrowing of the coronary arteries after the angioplasty and halved the chance that these blood vessels would close up again and require another angioplasty. High homocysteine levels can also make blood clot more easily than it should, increasing the risk of blood vessel blockages and stroke or heart attack.

Homocysteine is normally changed into other amino acids for use by the body. If your homocysteine level is too high, you may not have enough B vitamins to help this process. Most people with a high homocysteine level don't get enough folate (also called folic acid), vitamin B6 (pyridoxine), or vitamin B12 in their diet. Replacing these vitamins helps return homocysteine levels to normal. Other possible causes of a high homocysteine level include low levels of thyroid hormone, kidney disease, psoriasis, some medicines, or inherited deficiencies in the enzymes used to process homocysteine in the body.

HORMONES

ESTROGEN DEFICIENCY INDUCED BY MENOPAUSE

Six of ten studies showed that women who took estrogen had a lower risk for Alzheimer's disease. The best of these studies was the Baltimore Longitudinal Study of Aging, in which 472 women who were going through menopause or had completed it were followed for up to sixteen years. Women who never used estrogen during the study were twice as likely to develop dementia.

This study and others showing beneficial effects of estrogen have recently been contradicted by reports from the Women's Health Initiative, which found that women who used Premarin (an estrogen made from horse ovaries) were twice as likely to develop Alzheimer's as nonestrogen users. But the Women's Health Initiative study did not examine the risk of AD using forms of estrogen made by the human ovary, such as estradiol. Evidence suggesting that these more natural forms of estrogen for women may still reduce AD risk and provide other benefits comes from the largest study ever done on the severest form of estrogen deficiency—hysterectomy with removal of the ovaries. This study of a hundred thousand women who participated in the 1986 National Mortality Followback Survey found that women with a hysterectomy were twice as likely to develop dementia. What one can conclude from this complex maze of seemingly contradictory research findings is that women should avoid Premarin and other forms of estrogen that are not made by the human ovary. But severe reductions in female estrogen hormones are equally harmful and should be treated. A large body of basic scientific research demonstrates sound reasons why estrogen, in the right amount, protects the brain, the blood vessels, and the bones. Human forms of estrogen, taken in the smallest amounts needed to keep blood estradiol levels from falling too low after menopause, are reasonably safe and have not, to date, been demonstrated by the Women's Health Initiative or any other study to be harmful.

If you are a woman with a family history of dementia, then you should have a blood estradiol test after menopause to determine if you have estrogen deficiency. You can then evaluate with your doctor whether low-dose estradiol or other natural estrogens would be worth taking. The situation is more complex in women with a family history of both AD and breast or uterine cancer, because estrogen use increases the risk of these two cancers. Whether low-dose estradiol significantly increases the risk of heart disease or stroke in women without symptoms is more controversial. The relative benefits of taking low-dose estradiol after menopause (reduced risk of AD and osteoporosis) may be greater than the relative risks (increased risk of endometrial cancer, breast cancer, and maybe stroke and heart disease), but the decision regarding treatment depends on your personal history and risk factors for each of these diseases.

Although not all studies agree, estrogen use after menopause appears to significantly reduce AD risk. Estrogen use in estrogen-deficient women can also improve verbal fluency and possibly verbal short-term memory. Evista is a form of estrogen that is safer for women with increased risk of breast or uterine cancer.

TESTOSTERONE DEFICIENCY IN MALES

Testosterone levels normally start to decline after age fifty. By age eighty, testosterone levels are 20 to 50 percent of their former adult levels. Low testosterone levels may increase dementia risk. A case-control study involving 83 AD patients and 103 normal volunteers of similar age showed significantly reduced total testosterone levels in AD males. But until a well-designed group study is done, it is not certain whether testosterone deficiency is a risk factor for AD.

Men who have or have had prostate cancer treatment, or men fifty and older, may develop cognitive impairment due to testosterone deficiency, which can be checked by a blood test. Symptoms including difficulty with vision not due to eye problems, difficulty remembering locations or faces or other objects of interest, breast enlargement, or a change in the distribution of body hair should alert one to check for testosterone deficiency.

PARKINSON'S DISEASE

Parkinson's disease (PD) is caused by the loss of dopamine-producing cells. There is a significant connection between PD and AD. There is no known cure for PD, but with early detection there are medications that help with the symptoms. It has also been suggested that coenzyme Q10, a powerful antioxidant, along with high doses of vitamins C and E, may be helpful in delaying the need for stronger and stronger medications. Vitamin B6 increases the production of dopamine and may be helpful early in the disease process. The natural hormone melatonin, which regulates sleep, has been found to reduce tremors and protect against free radical damage on dopamine neurons. Fish oils and flaxseeds contain omega-3 fatty acids that have nerve-nourishing effects that can boost dopamine.

SEIZURES AND SEIZURE MEDICATION

About 125,000 Americans develop epilepsy every year. Thousands more experience isolated seizures that may or may not happen again in the future, but only recurring seizures are defined as epilepsy. Treatment of epilepsy has improved dramatically in recent years. Seizures can often be controlled, and the chances of long-term remission are improving all the time. But seizures and certain antiseizure medications can have a negative effect on brain function and be associated with dementia. During seizures there is dramatically increased brain activity, and then in the in-between period there is significant decreased activity. Antiseizure medications work by increasing inhibition in the brain. If this is done too enthusiastically, as with the older antiseizure medication like Dilantin and phenobarbital, the drug can cause overall decreased activity and damage the healthy cells around the seizure-promoting ones.

Obviously, seizure disorders must be vigorously treated. Once a person is two years seizure free, however, many neurologists start to taper off the antiseizure medications to see how much is needed. Also, newer antiseizure medications, such as Trileptal, are less likely to cause too much overall inhibition of brain function. If you are taking an antiseizure medication and notice memory problems, that is a symptom that the temporal lobes may be calmed too much. The most common cause of seizures in someone with epilepsy is not taking seizure medication as prescribed. For some people whose seizures cannot be controlled with medication, there is the option of surgery to remove the damaged tissue. Sometimes it is possible to identify a certain action or event that will always produce seizures in sensitive people. Seizure "triggers" include flickering lights, breathing very quickly and deeply, drinking an excessive amount of fluid, and even, in very rare cases, reading or listening to a certain piece of music. Sleep deprivation (like staying up all night studying) may produce seizures; so may excessive use of alcohol or withdrawal from certain drugs. Avoiding seizure triggers may require no more than a slight readjustment of activities.

SLEEP APNEA

Obstructive sleep apnea—a condition associated with loud snoring, stopping breathing entirely for brief periods many times during the night, and chronic tiredness—can cause cognitive impairment. The only brain SPECT study of obstructive sleep apnea examined fourteen moderate to severely affected patients, who stopped breathing more than thirty times per hour. Their brain SPECT scans showed significantly reduced activity in the left parietal lobe. Reduced left parietal lobe activity can impair comprehension, making it difficult to understand conversations or read books. Treatment of the sleep apnea with nasal Continuous Positive Airway Pressure (CPAP, a machine that pushes air at a high pressure through the nasal passageways) completely reversed the impaired brain activity in these patients. Sleep apnea should be evaluated and treated as early as possible.

SMOKING

Cigarette smoking accounts for 12 percent of all the strokes in the United States and is therefore a major risk factor for dementia. Smoking is also a risk for lung, stomach, and bladder cancer; hypertension; and heart disease. Nicotine constricts small blood vessels in all the organs of the body, including the brain, and prematurely ages everything.

Obviously, stop smoking. I know this is often much more easily said than done. Over the years I have helped many people stop smoking, and I have found that no one program works for everyone. Hypnosis is effective for some, the use of nicotine patches or gum works for others, the medication

Wellbutrin (buproprion), a dopamine-enhancing antidepressant, is helpful for others, and some respond to group therapy. In my experience it is usually a combination of treatments that are needed.

In order to keep your brain young, you need to keep your mind and body young as well. As you can see, the strategies are simple—stop polluting your body, eat good food, exercise your mind and body, and treat disease early. The following chapter will discuss rational supplementation as the next part of the program for keeping your brain young and making your good brain great.

SUPERCHARGING NEURONS

BRAIN-SPECIFIC SUPPLEMENTS

Most medical students are taught that people do not need vitamins and supplements. If you eat a balanced diet, they are told, you get all the nutrients needed. I was told this in medical school, and the mantra is still being disseminated twenty-seven years later. The one problem with this advice is that no one I know has a balanced diet. In the age of fast everything—food, information, communication—three nutritious meals a day are long gone. In addition, several antiaging supplements have been found to be helpful even if your diet is pretty good.

Having reviewed the medical research on prevention and supplementation, I take high-potency multiple vitamins every day, along with extra vitamins C and E, ginkgo biloba, alpha-lipoic acid, phosphatidal serine, acetyl-l-carnitine, CoQ10, and fish oil. Despite being a very busy physician, I also do my best to exercise daily for thirty minutes or more and try to eat right, including fish, fruit, and vegetables. These preventive actions are a part of my life because enough research supports the use of each of these strategies to have the best brain and body possible. Furthermore, these preventive strategies are safe if you are being monitored by your physician on a regular basis. People who have bleeding problems or take blood thinners need to exert caution with these recommendations and check with their doctor, especially with the recommendations for ginkgo and vitamin E. One of the keys to a great brain is to use prevention and supplementation strategies as early and wisely as possible.

Before discussing each of the supplements, it is important to discuss the pros and cons of using them. There are significant advantages to using proper brain supplementation, as well as a few downsides or controversies you need to know about.

The most significant benefit to using natural supplements is that they are geared to prevent illness rather than just treat it. Preventing problems is dramatically more cost effective than treating them after they have occurred. Engaging in supplement strategies helps build an attitude of prevention and hopefully leads to a healthier lifestyle overall. Waiting until you have an illness, such as a stroke or Alzheimer's disease, is *always* more expensive than spending time, effort, and money to prevent it. In addition, supplements are often very effective for mild to moderate problems, with fewer side effects than most pharmaceuticals. Compliance tends to be higher for these products, which means that people are more likely to take them over the long run. Generally, supplement strategies are less expensive than pharmaceutical alternatives. In addition, you never have to tell an insurance company that you have taken them. As awful as it sounds, taking prescription medication for brain problems, or even to enhance brain health, can affect a person's insurability. This is true for medications that treat anxiety, depression, bipolar disorder, ADD, and many other problems. I know many patients, colleagues, and friends who have been denied health or life insurance because of the medications they were taking. If there are natural alternatives, they are worth considering.

The supplement picture is not all rosy, and some of the disadvantages have to be considered. Even though supplements are generally less expensive than medications, they may be more expensive for you precisely because they are not covered by insurance. In addition, many people are unaware that natural supplements can have side effects. Just because a substance is natural does not mean it is innocuous. For example, St. John's wort, one of my favorite natural antidepressants that works like a mild form of Prozac in the brain, can cause sun sensitivity and can deactivate the effectiveness of other medications, such as birth control pills and antivirals.

One of the major issues of concern regarding natural products is the lack of standardization and quality control. Rigid quality control is not required for these products, and the manufacturing process has many variables. There are variables with the plant part used for herbs, such as age, ripeness when harvested, growing environment, and storage conditions. The therapeutic and toxic components of the supplement may vary considerably. There also may be issues with contamination. Different components of each herb can exhibit different pharmacological effects. It is critical to get brands you trust that have been tested and shown to be reliable. Another disadvantage is that people get a lot of their advice about supplements from the clerk at the grocery store, who may not have the most up-to-date information. I often send patients to www.consumerlabs.com, an independent laboratory that posts the results of quality control tests.

Even given the cons, supplements, to my mind, are worth serious consideration. We can be targeted and thoughtful in our choices, and we can find dedicated companies that produce high-quality products. It amazes me how many physicians have a knee-jerk negative reaction to supplements despite the large amounts of research on them. I teach the course on supplements to the psychiatric residents at the University of California at Irvine. Many of the residents start the course with a negative attitude about them; invariably one will say there is not enough research on them and that they do not really contain the ingredients on the labels. At the end of the course, when they have learned about the extensive research and good-quality companies, many of the young psychiatrists are excited about the possibility of using supplements to help their patients, and many even start to take the ones I discuss below. I have had enough personal experience with the side effects of pharmaceuticals to believe that patients deserve to know about natural alternatives.

The rest of the chapter explores some of my favorite brain supplementation strategies. You do not need to take all of them. Evaluate each product for your own personal situation and risk factors. Unless you have a reason not to, I believe everyone should engage in regular mental and physical exercise and take a multiple vitamin, vitamin C, and fish oil every day. After age forty, when cellular energy production and antioxidant levels in the body naturally are lower, most people will also benefit from acetyl-L-carnitine, alpha-lipoic acid, and CoQ10.

ACETYL-L-CARNITINE

Acetyl-L-carnitine (ALC) has been reported to improve mental focus, enhance energy, and slow aging. Research has shown that ALC increases levels of neurotransmitters needed for memory, focus, and learning, and repairs the damage done to brain cells caused by stress and poor nutrition.

About 95 percent of energy production in your cells occurs in the mitochondria. Many diseases of aging are increasingly being referred to as "mitochondrial disorders." ALC has been shown to help increase energy production in the mitochondria.

Some people report feeling an increase in mental energy and focus within twenty minutes of taking ALC, so you should not take it late in the day, as it may give you insomnia. Even though ALC is not a stimulant, it seems to naturally increase energy in the brain. Over thirty studies show that ALC slows or prevents age-related decline in mental function. In one study 1.5 g of ALC given to 236 older adults each day for forty-five days significantly increased the effectiveness of performance on all the measures of cognitive functioning, memory, and constructional thinking. Twenty adults given 1.5 g of ALC experienced a reversal of many of the signs of brain aging. Alcoholics with cognitive impairment have also benefited from ALC. Acetyl-L-carnitine is potentially valuable in helping depression. One hundred sixty patients who had suffered from a stroke a year or more ago were given 1.5 g of ALC a day for eight weeks. This led to increased speed of recovery, as well as improved mood and attention span. A total of more than six hundred patients with Alzheimer's have been studied in over twenty years of research, demonstrating that ALC benefits patients with dementia.

Because of a lack of long-term safety studies, ALC is not advised for pregnant women or nursing mothers. Mild gastrointestinal symptoms may occur in those taking ALC, including nausea, vomiting, abdominal cramps, and diarrhea. Increased agitation has been reported in some with Alzheimer's disease when taking oral ALC. In people with seizure disorders, an increase in seizure frequency has been reported after taking ALC.

You should consider ALC if you suffer from tiredness, mental fatigue, memory loss, or attentional problems. The typical dose is 500 to 1,500 mg a day.

ALPHA-LIPOIC ACID

Alpha-lipoic acid (ALA) is an antioxidant that increases the potency of many other antioxidants, including vitamins C and E and, most importantly, glutathione. Glutathione is the most powerful antioxidant in cells and acts to regulate the cells' ability to absorb free radicals and prevent damage, which has been demonstrated in studies in blood, skeletal muscle, and liver cells. ALA is a small molecule that readily enters the brain to protect it from free radical damage. ALA helps to prevent some of the diseases that put the brain at risk for problems ranging from cancer to AIDS. It has shown significant benefits with varying levels of scientific support. In one study ALA reduced the size of strokes by as much as 50 percent. There is evidence that it may help prevent or slow the development of atherosclerosis (hardening of the arteries). Remember, whatever is good for the heart is good for the brain. Researchers demonstrated in a sixteen-week trial that ALA in oral doses of 600 mg daily for eight weeks significantly improved levels of LDL-cholesterol in healthy human subjects. ALA appears to slow aging of the brain through its potent antioxidant properties.

Because of lack of long-term safety data, alpha-lipoic acid should be avoided by pregnant women and nursing mothers. Those with diabetes and problems with glucose intolerance are cautioned that ALA may lower blood glucose levels. Blood glucose should be monitored and antidiabetic drug doses adjusted, if necessary, to avoid possible low blood sugar states. In doses up to 600 mg a day no side effects have been noted.

You should consider taking ALA if you are over forty and are at risk for dementia or other memory problems, cancer, or stroke. The typical dose is 100 to 200 mg a day.

COENZYME Q10 (COQ10)

Coenzyme Q10 (CoQ10), also known as ubiquinone, is a powerful antioxidant discovered by researchers at the University of Wisconsin in 1957. The name of this supplement comes from the word *ubiquitous,* which means "found everywhere." Indeed, CoQ10 is found in every cell in the body. CoQ10 is an enzyme that lives inside the mitochondria of your cells and helps convert oxygen into usable energy. Organs that use a lot of oxygen are the heart, muscles, kidneys, pancreas, and brain. If the mitochondria of these oxygen-demanding organs do not properly convert oxygen into energy, they can be damaged. Japanese scientists first discovered the therapeutic properties of CoQ10 in the 1960s. Today it is widely prescribed in Europe, Israel, and Japan for heart conditions. CoQ10 appears to assist the heart during times of stress on the heart muscle, perhaps by helping it use energy more efficiently.

Certain cholesterol-lowering drugs, known as statins, significantly lower levels of CoQ10. This may be particularly hazardous for patients with heart disease, suggesting a possible indication for CoQ10 in many, if not all, individuals using these cholesterol-lowering drugs. There is also some evidence that CoQ10 might boost energy and speed recovery of exercise-related muscle exhaustion and damage.

Recently, it was discovered that mutations in a gene on chromosome 4 produce Parkinson's disease (PD), a movement disorder that affects about one percent of all people over fifty years old. This gene helps regulate the activity of CoQ10 in the mitochondria. In people with PD, CoQ10 activity is reduced in the basal ganglia, therefore causing problems with movement. Furthermore, reduced CoQ10 blood levels are found in people with Lewy Body dementia, a more widespread form of PD. A recent multicenter trial of eighty people with early-stage untreated PD examined the effect of a placebo versus 300, 600, or 1,200 mg of CoQ10 per day for eighteen months. CoQ10 delayed the progression of PD symptoms by 44 percent, and 1,200 mg per day slowed the decline in movement better than lower doses. CoQ10 may be a safe and effective way to delay the severely debilitating movement disorder PD. People with PD or Lewy Body disease, or a positive family history of these disorders, should consider taking CoQ10. If symptoms are already present, then 1,200 mg per day is an effective dose. In people without symptoms, lower doses are probably effective, but the exact dose is not established.

There has been one report of CoQ10 decreasing the effectiveness of the medication warfarin. Those taking it should be aware of this possibility. Because of lack of long-term safety studies, pregnant women and nursing mothers should avoid CoQ10 supplements. Clinical reports suggest that CoQ10 may lower blood sugar levels in diabetics, so they should be made aware of this possibility and monitored as needed. Mild intestinal symptoms such as nausea and diarrhea have been reported, particularly with higher doses (200 mg or more daily).

CoQ10 is available in different formulations: oil-based capsules, powder-filled capsules, and tablets and solubilized softgels (microemulsions and others). The solubilized softgels are claimed to give higher absorption. CoQ10 is best taken with food. The typical dosage is 30 to 200 mg per day.

OMEGA-3 FATTY ACIDS

Fish oils, also known as marine oils, are fats found in fish, particularly cold-water fish, and other marine life such as phytoplankton and krill. These oils are rich sources of long-chain polyunsaturated fatty acids, also called omega-3 fatty acids. The two most studied fish oils are eicosapentaenoic acid (EPA) and docosahexaenoic acid (DHA). DHA is a vital component of cell membranes, especially those in the brain and retina. Supplemental fish oils have been shown to have many positive effects on the body. They lower triglyceride levels and have anti-inflammatory, antiarrhythmic, immune-enhancing, and nerve-cell-stabilizing properties. In addition, they help to maintain normal blood flow as they lower the body's ability to form clots. DHA is vital for normal brain development for the fetus and infant and for the maintenance of normal brain function throughout life. DHA appears to be a major factor in the fluidity and flexibility of brain cell membranes. It could play a major role in maintaining how we think and feel. Fish oils appear to have mood-stabilizing properties when used in the treatment of bipolar disorder. On SPECT scans bipolar disorder shows overall increased activity in the brain, and EPA and DHA tend to calm or dampen these over-active brain signals.

A four-month double-blind, placebo-controlled study of thirty subjects with bipolar disorder compared the effects of fish oil supplements with a placebo. Fourteen subjects received 9.6 g daily of fish oil, consisting of 6.2 g of EPA and 3.4 grams of DHA, and sixteen subjects received olive oil as a placebo. This study showed improvement in the short-term course of the disorder with fish oil supplementation. Among those taking fish oil, longer periods of remission were observed in nearly every outcome category, and the results were statistically significant. Mild gastrointestinal side effects were reported in the fish oil group.

In a landmark study published in the journal *Lancet*, researchers examined the effect of dietary fish oil and vitamin E supplementation on death and disease in more than eleven thousand subjects who had suffered a heart attack within three months of entering the trial. The trial lasted for forty-two months. The most significant result was the reduction in risk for overall and sudden cardiac death, which it is believed was due to the antiarrythmic effect of the fish oil. The study suggests that up to twenty lives per thousand post–heart attack patients could be saved by consuming daily doses of less than 1 g of EPA and DHA.

An analysis of seventeen studies with fish oil indicates that supplementation with 3 or more g of fish oil daily can lead to clinically relevant blood pressure reductions in individuals with untreated hypertension, although it did not lower blood pressure in those who were normal. An analysis of another group of studies on the effect of fish oil following coronary angioplasty indicates that subjects who had undergone successful angioplasty had a significantly lower rate (13.9 percent) of recurrent problems when given 4 to 5 g daily of mixtures of EPA and DHA for three months to one year following the angioplasty. What's good for your heart is also good for your brain.

Fish oil supplements have many other physical benefits. Daily use of fish oil of at least 3 g of EPA and DHA mixtures for a period of twelve weeks or longer has been found to reduce the number of tender joints and the amount of morning stiffness in people with rheumatoid arthritis, to the extent that they were reported to have lowered or discontinued use of nonsteroidal anti-inflammatory drugs or other antirheumatic drugs. The supplements appeared to be well tolerated in these individuals, and no serious side effects were reported.

Because of the possible anticlotting effect of fish oil supplements, hemophiliacs and those taking warfarin (Coumadin) should exercise caution in their use. Fish oil supplements should be stopped before any surgical procedure. Diabetics who take fish oil supplements should be monitored by their physicians. There have been no reports of serious adverse events in those taking fish oil supplements, even up to 15 g daily for prolonged periods of time. The side effects that have been reported include mild gastrointestinal upsets such as nausea and diarrhea, halitosis, burping and "fishy"-smelling breath, skin, and even urine. The blood-thinning effects can cause occasional nosebleeds and easy bruising.

I have several favorite sources of fish oil supplementation. One is a supplement called Coromega, made by European Reference Botanical Laboratories; see www.coromega.com for information. Coromega is a high-quality supplement that gives the right ratio of EPA to DHA, and it tastes great. Often fish oil supplements leave a fishy taste, but Coromega tastes like orange pudding, and we can even get children to take it without a fuss. Also, Dr. René Thomas has made a spearmint-flavored fish oil, as well as a healthy ice cream called Nature's Might Bites (www.kidsneedusnow.org) that contains high doses of omega-3 fatty acids. The wonderful thing is that the ice cream also contains high levels of high-quality protein and is not filled with empty calories. Life is good when you can get your fish oil supplement in orange pudding or ice cream. In addition, Dr. Sears (www.drsears.com) makes a high-quality fish oil product, as do Nordic Naturals and Omega Brite.

The typical dosage of fish oil is 1 to 2 g a day for prevention and 4 to 6 g a day to treat illness. High-quality fish oil can be taken by pregnant women and has been shown to help their moods when prone to bipolar disorder. But make sure it is high quality and does not contain any contaminants.

GINKGO BILOBA

The prettiest brains I have seen are those on ginkgo. Ginkgo biloba, from the Chinese ginkgo tree, is a powerful antioxidant that is best known for its ability to enhance circulation, memory, and concentration. The best-studied form of ginkgo biloba is a special extract called EBg 761, which has been studied in blood vessel disease, clotting disorders, depression, and Alzheimer's disease. A comparison in 2000 of all the published placebo-controlled studies longer than six months for ginkgo biloba extract EGb 761 versus Cognex, Aricept, and Exelon showed they all had similar benefits for mild to moderate AD patients.

The most widely publicized U.S. study of ginkgo biloba was done by Dr. P. L. Le Bars and colleagues from the New York Institute for Medical Research, which appeared in the *Journal of the American Medical Association* in 1997. EGb 761 was used to assess the efficacy and safety in treating Alzheimer's disease and vascular dementia. It was a fifty-two-week multicenter study with patients who had mild to severe symptoms. Patients were randomly assigned to treatment with EGb 761 (120 mg/d) or a placebo. Progress was monitored at 12, 26, and 52 weeks, and 202 patients finished the study. At the end of the study the authors concluded that EGb was safe and that it appeared capable of stabilizing and, in a substantial number of cases, improving the cognitive performance and social functioning of demented patients for six months to one year. Although modest, the changes induced by EGb were objectively measured and were of sufficient magnitude to be recognized by the caregivers.

Consider taking ginkgo if you are at risk for memory problems or stroke or suffer from low energy or decreased concentration. There are many different forms of ginkgo, making dosing confusing. In the U.S., Ginkoba and Ginkgold (Nature's Way) are brands that have been compounded to reflect EGb 761. The usual effective dose is 60 to 120 mg twice a day. There is a small risk of bleeding in the body, and the dosages of other blood-thinning agents being taken may sometimes have to be reduced.

PHOSPHATIDYLSERINE

Phosphatidylserine (PS) is a naturally occurring nutrient that is found in foods such as fish, green leafy vegetables, soy products, and rice. It is a component of cell membranes. There are reports of the potential of PS to help improve age-related declines in memory, learning, verbal skills, and concentration. PET studies of patients who have taken PS show that it produces a general increase in metabolic activity in the brain. In the largest multicenter study to date of phosphatidylserine and Alzheimer's disease, 142 subjects aged forty to eighty were given 200 mg of phosphatidylserine per day or a placebo over a three-month period. Those treated with phosphatidylserine exhibited improvement on several items on the scales normally used to assess Alzheimer's status. The differences between the placebo and experimental groups were small but statistically significant. Effective doses of PS have been reported to be 300 mg per day. The types of symptoms that have improved in placebo-controlled studies of cognitive impairment or dementia include loss of interest, reduced activities, social isolation, anxiety, memory, concentration, and recall. Milder stages of impairment tend to respond to PS better than more severe stages. With regard to depression in elderly individuals, Dr. M. Maggioni and his colleagues studied the effects of oral PS (300 mg per day) versus a placebo and noted significant improvements in mood, memory, and motivation after thirty days of PS treatment.

The typical dose of PS is 100 to 300 mg a day.

L-THEANINE

L-theanine is an amino acid mainly found naturally in the green tea plant. L-theanine is the predominant amino acid in green tea and makes up 50 percent of the total free amino acids in the plant. L-theanine is considered the main component responsible for the taste of green tea. It is marketed in Japan as a nutritional supplement for mood modulation. L-theanine may also have activity in modulating the metabolism of cancer chemotherapeutic agents and ameliorating their side effects.

L-theanine has been shown to penetrate the brain and produce significant increases in concentrations of the neurotransmitters serotonin and dopamine. These findings led to recent studies investigating the possibility that L-theanine might enhance learning ability, induce relaxation, and relieve emotional stress. Memory and learning ability were said to be improved in young male Wistar rats given 180 mg of L-theanine daily for four months. Human performance was assessed using a test for learning ability and passive and active avoidance tests for memory. The mental effects of L-theanine were tested in a small group of volunteers divided into two groups, defined as "high-anxiety" and "low-anxiety" groups. The volunteers were females aged eighteen to twenty-two. Their level of anxiety was assessed by a manifest anxiety scale. Subjects received water, 50 mg of L-theanine, or 200 mg of L-theanine solution once a week. Brain waves were measured 60 minutes after administration. The 200 mg dose (dissolved in 100 ml of water) resulted in significantly greater production of alpha waves than was observed in subjects receiving water. The effect was dose-dependent. The researchers regarded the significantly increased production of alpha-brain-wave activity as an index of increased relaxation.

Pregnant women and nursing mothers should avoid L-theanine supplements. Use of L-theanine supplements concomitantly with cancer chemotherapeutic agents must be done under medical supervision. There are no known adverse reactions.

L-theanine supplements are available for the promotion of relaxation and the modulation of mood. Doses used are between 50 and 200 mg, as necessary. L-theanine is available in some green tea preparations. The amino acid constitutes between 1 and 2 percent of the dry weight of green tea leaves.

VINPOCETINE

Vinpocetine is not for everyone, but it does seem to help people at risk for heart disease or stroke. It also helps lower high homocysteine levels, which are dangerous to your heart and brain. Vinpocetine is derived from an extract of the common periwinkle plant (*Vinca minor*) and is used in Europe, Japan, and Mexico as a pharmaceutical agent for the treatment of blood vessel disease in the brain and cognitive disorders. In the United States, it is available as a dietary supplement. It is sometimes called a nootropic (meaning "cognition enhancer," from the Greek *noos*, "mind"). Vinpocetine selectively widens arteries and capillaries, increasing blood flow to the brain. It also combats the accumulation of platelets in the blood, improving circulation. Because of these properties, vinpocetine was first used in the treatment of cerebrovascular disorders and acute memory loss due to late-life dementia. But it also has a beneficial effect on memory problems associated with normal aging.

Vinpocetine may be useful for a wide variety of brain problems. A 1976 study found that vinpocetine immediately increased circulation in fifty people with abnormal blood flow. After one month of taking moderate doses of vinpocetine, patients showed improvement on memorization tests. After a prolonged period of vinpocetine treatment, cognitive impairment diminished significantly or disappeared altogether in many of the patients. A 1987 study of elderly patients with chronic cerebral dysfunction found that patients who took vinpocetine performed better on psychological evaluations after the ninety-day trial period than did those who received a placebo. More recent studies have shown that vinpocetine reduces neural damage and protects against oxidative damage from harmful beta-amyloid buildup. In a multicenter, double-blind, placebo-controlled study lasting sixteen weeks, 203 patients described as having mild-to-moderate memory problems, including primary dementia, were treated with varying doses of vinpocetine or a placebo. Significant improvement was achieved in the vinpocetine-treated group as measured by "global improvement" and cognitive performance scales. Three 10 mg doses daily were as effective as or more effective than three 20 mg doses daily. Similarly good results were found in another double-blind clinical trial testing vinpocetine versus a placebo in elderly patients with blood vessel and central nervous system degenerative disorders. Some preliminary research suggests that vinpocetine may also have protective effects on both sight and hearing.

Reported adverse reactions include nausea, dizziness, insomnia, drowsiness, dry mouth, transient hypotension, transient fast heart rate, pressure headaches, and facial flushing. Slight reductions in both systolic and diastolic blood pressure with prolonged use of vinpocetine have been reported, as well as slight reductions in blood sugar levels.

The usual dosage is 10 mg a day.

MULTIPLE VITAMINS

Due to our poor diets, I recommend that all of my patients take a high-quality 100 percent multiple vitamin every day. Over the last twenty years, our understanding of the benefits of vitamins has rapidly advanced, and it now appears that people who get enough vitamins may be able to help prevent such common chronic illnesses as cancer, heart disease, dementia, and osteoporosis, according to Drs. Robert Fletcher and Kathleen Fairfield of Harvard University, who wrote the guidelines for vitamins published in the *Journal of the American Medical Association* (*JAMA*) in 2002. The last time *JAMA* made a comprehensive review of vitamins, about twenty years before, it concluded that people of normal health shouldn't take multivitamins because they were a waste of time and money. People can get all the nutrients they need from their diet, *JAMA* advised, adding that only pregnant women and chronically sick people might need certain vitamins. That was at a time when knowledge about vitamins was just beginning to expand. The role that low levels of folate, or folic acid, play in neural tube defects, for instance, was unknown, as was its role as a major risk factor for heart disease. Almost 80 percent of Americans do not eat at least five helpings of fruits and vegetables a day, the recommended minimum amount believed to provide sufficient essential nutrients. Humans do not make their own vitamins, except for some vitamin D, so they must get them from an outside source to prevent problems.

B VITAMINS

B vitamins play an integral role in the functioning of the nervous system, and they help the brain synthesize neurotransmitters that affect mood and thinking. A balanced complex of the B vitamins is essential for energy and for balancing hormone levels. Folate and B12 deficiencies are well-known causes of cognitive impairment or dementia as well as coronary heart disease. They can also elevate homocysteine levels, which increase risks for stroke, heart disease, and Alzheimer's disease. Patients deficient in folate can show significant improvements in memory and attention when treated with folic acid for as few as sixty days. In addition to having a direct effect, B vitamins indirectly impact mental function by altering the levels of harmful or beneficial substances in the body. For instance, elevated homocysteine (an amino acid) levels have been linked to heart disease and poorer cognitive function. A combination therapy with B vitamins—folate and vitamins B12 and B6—is an effective means to reduce elevated homocysteine levels. To maintain low plasma homocysteine concentration, people should be advised to increase their consumption of eggs, green leafy vegetables, and fruits, which are all rich in B vitamins.

Another study showed that less-than-optimal levels of vitamin B6, B12, and folic acid lead to a deficiency of S-adenosylmethionine (SAMe). SAMe deficiency can cause depression, dementia, or a degeneration of the nerves. The typical American diet does not always provide these essential vitamins, at least in high doses. Because B vitamins are water soluble and are excreted from the body daily, they must be replenished on a regular basis. Older people are at greater risk for vitamin deficiency because they tend to eat less of a variety of foods, and their requirements for certain vitamins such as B6 are actually higher. Older people may also have problems with efficient nutrient absorption from food. Even healthy older people often exhibit deficiencies in vitamin B6, vitamin B12, and folate.

B6 supplementation has been found to be helpful for memory function. Dr. J. B. Deijen and colleagues from Holland found in a study of seventy-six elderly males that giving vitamin B6 versus a placebo improved memory function.

Take 100 percent of the B vitamins every day. Make sure you take at least 400 mcg of folate and 500 mcg of B12 a day.

VITAMIN C

Unlike most mammals, humans do not have the ability to make their own vitamin C (ascorbic acid). Therefore we must obtain it through our diet or supplementation. Vitamin C is required for the synthesis of collagen, an important structural component of blood vessels, tendons, ligaments, and bone. Vitamin C also plays an important role in the synthesis of the neurotransmitter norepinephrine. Neurotransmitters are critical to brain function and are known to affect mood. In addition, vitamin C is required for the synthesis of carnitine, a small molecule that is essential for the transport of fat to cellular organelles called mitochondria, for conversion to energy. Vitamin C is also a highly effective antioxidant. Even in small amounts, vitamin C can protect proteins, fats, carbohydrates, and DNA from damage by free radicals. Vitamin C also helps to recycle other antioxidants, such as vitamin E.

Low or deficient intake of vitamin C is associated with an increased risk of cardiovascular diseases, and modest dietary intakes of about 100 mg per day in some studies were sufficient for reduction of cardiovascular disease risk among nonsmoking men and women. With respect to vitamin C and strokes, a prospective study that followed more than two thousand residents of a rural Japanese community for twenty years found that the risk of stroke in those with the highest serum levels of vitamin C was 29 percent lower than in those with the lowest serum levels of vitamin C. Additionally, the risk of stroke in those who consumed vegetables six to seven days a week was 54 percent lower than in those who consumed vegetables zero to two days a week. In this population, serum levels of vitamin C were highly correlated with fruit and vegetable intakes. A number of studies have also investigated the role of vitamin C in cancer prevention. Most have shown that higher intakes of vitamin C are associated with decreased incidence of cancers of the mouth, throat and vocal cords, esophagus, stomach, colon-rectum, and lung. A ten-year Rotterdam study of 5,395 individuals fifty-five years and older showed that high dietary intake of vitamins C and E (fruits and vegetables) reduces the risk of Alzheimer's disease by about 20 percent.

As shown in the following table, different fruits and vegetables vary in their vitamin C content, but five servings should average out to at least 200 mg of vitamin C.

Food	Serving	Vitamin C (mg)
Orange juice	¾ cup (6 ounces)	75
Grapefruit juice	¾ cup (6 ounces)	60
Orange	1 medium	70
Grapefruit	½ medium	44
Strawberries	1 cup, whole	82
Tomato	1 medium	23
Sweet red pepper	½ cup, raw chopped	141
Broccoli	½ cup, cooked	58
Potato	1 medium, baked	26

Side effects are rare but can occasionally include urinary tract infections due to acidification. Vitamin C is available in many forms, but there is little scientific evidence that any one form is better absorbed or more effective than another. I recommend a vitamin C intake of 250 mg twice a day for adults. Consuming at least five servings of fruits and vegetables daily may provide about 200 mg of vitamin C. Most multivitamin supplements provide 60 mg of vitamin C.

VITAMIN E

Vitamin E is an oil-soluble vitamin that is found in oils, nuts, and seeds. It is considered to be an antioxidant vitamin. Large doses will act as an anticoagulant or blood thinner. The Recommended Daily Allowance (RDA) for vitamin E is about 20 I.U. per day. There are different forms of vitamin E, including gamma-tocopherol and the better-known alpha-tocopherol. The RDA was set for alpha-tocopherol. Artificial dl-alpha-tocopherol is considered to be only half as active as natural vitamin E. The gamma-tocopherol form of vitamin E may have even more potent physiological benefits.

Vitamin E has seen controversy in recent years. It has been reported to be a possible protective factor in dementia. In very high doses of 1,000 I.U. twice a day in people who already have symptoms of AD, it has been shown to delay AD's progression by one year. With regard to prevention in normal aging individuals, a recent three-year longitudinal study of 2,889 community residents 65 to 102 years old examined the influence of dietary and supplemental intake of vitamins C, E, and beta-carotene on the course of a variety of mental skills. The researchers tested working memory, short-term memory, overall mental ability, and complex task performance. They found that vitamin E, in doses of 400 I.U. per day or higher, resulted in a 36 percent reduction in the rate of cognitive decline, compared to subjects taking the lowest amount of vitamin E. Vitamin C and beta-carotene taken separately showed no effect. This is the first clinical trial evidence that vitamin E delays the onset of decline in mental skills in normal aging individuals. After an average follow-up of six years, 197 participants developed dementia, of which 146 had Alzheimer's. When adjustments were made for age, sex, alcohol intake, education, smoking habits, presence of carotid plaques, and use of antioxidative supplements, high intake of vitamin C and vitamin E was associated with a 20 percent lower risk of AD. Among current smokers, this relationship was most pronounced. The associations did not vary by education or by apolipoprotein E genotype.

A recent study published in the *Annals of Internal Medicine* stated that high doses of vitamin E are dangerous and should be avoided. This study considered doses of vitamin E in excess of 400 I.U. per day to be high and those less than 400 I.U. per day to be low. A recent study by Dr. E. Miller is an analysis of death rates in study populations gleaned from nineteen different research projects that included vitamin E use. The studies included vitamin E as a potential treatment for, or means of prevention of, various diseases, such as heart disease, Alzheimer's disease, and cataracts. In order for the research populations to be included in this study, each project had to have patients take vitamin E for at least one year, and each study had to have at least ten deaths during or after the time of the study.

The results, according to Dr. Miller, show that lower doses of vitamin E may be slightly protective for death, but that higher doses may slightly increase a patient's risk of death. He concluded that vitamin E used in high doses is dangerous. But there were a number of potential problems with the study. It analyzed several studies involving the use of vitamin E for various diseases, but it did not include some studies that have shown a correlation between vitamin E use and a reduced risk of coronary disease. Other potential problems that could confound the results of this study include the following:

- Vitamin E was often used in combination with pharmaceutical drugs being studied; the effects of these combinations were not discussed in the research.

- The populations being studied mostly consisted of elderly people with chronic diseases. The study recognizes this as a possible confounder, because elderly, sick people are more likely to be taking high doses of vitamin E. It would not be possible to generalize the findings to a young and healthy population.

- The study looked at different types of research studies that used different protocols and procedures, such as different doses of vitamin E taken for different lengths of time.

- The original studies didn't necessarily differentiate between natural and synthetic vitamin E.

- Some of the results of the original studies have been questioned.

Given the myriad positive studies with vitamin E, I still recommend it. Until further studies are performed, I recommend taking lower doses, in the neighborhood of 200 I.U. a day.

The kind of vitamin E you take matters. Mixed tocopherols, including alpha and gamma, seem to be more effective than alpha-tocopherol alone.

Alpha-tocopherol is the most common form sold in stores. Because of the relatively short duration of action of the tocopherols (two to four hours), taking them twice a day gives better cellular protection to your brain and body. Major sources of vitamin E in the American diet include vegetable oils (olive, sunflower, and safflower), nuts, whole grains, and green leafy vegetables.

Food	Serving	Alpha-tocopherol (mg)	Gamma-tocopherol (mg)
Olive oil	1 tablespoon	1.9	0.1
Soybean oil	1 tablespoon	1.2	10.8
Corn oil	1 tablespoon	1.9	8.2
Canola oil	1 tablespoon	2.4	4.2
Safflower oil	1 tablespoon	4.6	0.1
Sunflower oil	1 tablespoon	5.6	0.7
Almonds	1 ounce	7.3	0.3
Hazelnuts	1 ounce	4.3	0
Peanuts	1 ounce	2.4	2.4
Spinach	½ cup, raw chopped	1.8	0
Carrots	½ cup, raw chopped	0.4	0
Avocado (California)	1 medium	3.4	0.6

Vitamin E stabilizes lipid membranes in the brain and protects the brain from damage due to free radical formation in cells. It is known that antioxidant mechanisms decline with aging, so supplementation may be protective. Furthermore, taking vitamin C, such as 250 to 500 mg, with each dose of vitamin E improves the absorption of E into the brain. Although not yet tested in clinical trials, this probably improves the effect of vitamin E on delaying decline in mental skills.

Vitamin E side effects are rare. But vitamin E may affect anticoagulation levels for people on Coumadin and may affect cholesterol levels. People who take both vitamin E and Coumadin should have regular laboratory studies to check for any bleeding problems. People who take vitamin E and also have high cholesterol should have their fasting lipid panel monitored about every three to six months to determine the effect of vitamin E on cholesterol.

Table 1

HEALTHY BRAIN SUPPLEMENT STRATEGIES REVIEWED

Supplement	Effect	Dosage	Notes
Acetyl-L-carnitine (ALC)	Enhances cellular energy; increases acetylcholine; helps with neurological and heart issues	500–1,500 mg a day	For all adults, take daily
Alpha-lipoic acid (ALA)	Antioxidant; also increases potency of other antioxidants; helps with diabetes, stroke, some cancers; helps eliminate heavy metals from body	100–200 mg a day	For all adults, take daily
Coenzyme Q10 (CoQ10)	Antioxidant; increases cellular energy; helps with congestive heart failure; lowers cholesterol; may help with Parkinson's disease	30–200 mg a day	Use if at risk for heart disease or Parkinson's disease; solubilized softgels are claimed to give higher absorption; best taken with food
Fish oil (Omega-3 fatty acids)	Lower triglyceride levels; anti-inflammatory, anti-arrhythmic, immune-enhancing, and nerve-cell-stabilizing effect; also may enhance mood stability	1–2 g a day for prevention, 4–6 g to treat illness	For all adults and children, EPA/DHA ratio of 1.8 to 2 seems best; take pharmaceutical grade; due to anticlotting effect, hemophiliacs and those taking blood thinners should exercise caution in use

Ginkgo biloba	Antioxidant; enhances circulation; helps with memory problems, heart disease, high blood pressure, stroke	60–120 mg twice a day	For adults at risk for dementia, heart disease, or stroke; due to anticlotting effect, hemophiliacs and those taking blood thinners should exercise caution in use
Phosphatidylserine	Component of nerve cell membranes; increases metabolic brain activity; helps with mood, mild cognitive problems, and early Alzheimer's disease	100–300 mg a day	Use if at risk for dementia or memory problems
L-Theanine	Active ingredient in green tea; may increase serotonin and dopamine; may increase alpha-wave (relaxation) production	50–200 mg a day	May also drink 2 cups of green tea a day
Vinpocetine	Widens arteries and capillaries, increasing blood flow to the brain; helps with memory	10 mg a day	Use if you have high homocysteine levels or are at risk for heart disease or stroke; watch for dizziness or facial flushing, as it increases blood flow
Multiple vitamin	Helps balance our frequently poor diets	100 percent taken daily	For all, take daily

HEALTHY BRAIN SUPPLEMENT STRATEGIES REVIEWED (*cont.*)

Supplement	Effect	Dosage	Notes
Vitamin B	Helps brain synthesize neurotransmitters that affect mood and thinking; essential for neuronal health; helps lower harmful homocysteine levels, especially B6, B12, and folate	B complex; make sure it has 400–800 mcg folate, 50 mg of B6, and 500–1,000 mcg of B12	For all, take daily; can be part of a high-potency multiple vitamin
Vitamin C (ascorbic acid)	Powerful antioxidant that helps recycle Vitamin E; helps in risk reduction for Alzheimer's disease	250 mg twice a day	For all, take daily
Vitamin E (mixed tocopherols)	Powerful antioxidant that stabilizes cell membranes; helps in risk reduction for Alzheimer's disease, heart attack, stroke, and cancer	100 I.U. twice a day	For all, take daily; do not take dl-alpha form (*dl* stands for "don't like"); due to anticlotting effect, hemophiliacs and those taking blood thinners should exercise caution in use

* Note half dosage for children

STRESS

During times of stress other supplements or herbs might also be useful. Here are some I commonly recommend.

GABA

Gamma-aminobutyric acid (GABA) is an amino acid that also functions as a neurotransmitter in the brain. GABA is reported in the herbal literature to work in much the same way as the antianxiety drugs and the anticonvulsants. It helps stabilize nerve cells by decreasing their tendency to fire erratically or excessively. This means it has a calming effect for people who struggle with temper, irritability, and anxiety, whether these symptoms relate to anxiety or to temporal lobe disturbance. GABA can be taken as a supplement in doses ranging from 250 to 1,500 mg daily for adults and from 125 to 750 mg daily for children. For best effect, GABA should be taken in two or three divided doses.

S-ADENOSYLMETHIONINE (SAMe)

SAMe is involved with the production of several neurotransmitters. The brain normally manufactures all the SAMe it needs from the amino acid methionine. When a person is depressed, the synthesis of SAMe from methionine is impaired. SAMe is one of the best natural antidepressants, and in a number of recent studies, it has performed as well as conventional antidepressant medications. SAMe has been found to increase the neurotransmitters that are low when people have depression. I frequently recommend SAMe to people who suffer from fibromyalgia, a chronic muscle pain disorder. Fibromyalgia is very commonly complicated by anxiety and depression. *People who have bipolar disorder or manic-depressive illness should not take SAMe.* There have been a number of reported cases of SAMe causing manic or hypomanic episodes (excessively up or happy moods, extreme impulsivity in sexuality or spending money, pressured speech, and decreased need for sleep). SAMe should be taken in doses of 200 to 400 mg two to four times a day, and children should take half this amount. One of the problems with SAMe is its cost. Because many insurance companies do not cover herbal or supplemental treatments, SAMe is more expensive than prescription medication for some people. As it becomes a more popular intervention, the cost of SAMe may decrease.

ST. JOHN'S WORT

I have seen dramatic improvement for many of my patients on St. John's wort, and I have SPECT scan studies of patients before and after treatment with St. John's wort that document its effectiveness. This flowering herb is named after Saint John the Baptist because it blooms around June 24, his feast day, and because the red ring around the crushed flowers is a reminder of the blood of the beheaded saint. St. John's wort may be the most potent of all the supplements at increasing serotonin availability in the brain. The starting dosage is 300 mg a day for children, 300 mg twice a day for teens, and 600 mg in the morning and 300 mg at night for adults. Sometimes the dose may be slowly increased to 1,800 mg for adults. It is extremely important that the preparation of St. John's wort contain 0.3 percent hypericin, which is believed to be the active ingredient. St. John's wort decreases anterior cingulate gyrus hyperactivity for many patients and decreases moodiness. An unfortunate side effect is that it can also decrease prefrontal cortex activity. One of the women in the study said, "I'm happier, but I'm dingier." St. John's wort may make people more vulnerable to sunburn, and so extra sun protection is needed by anyone using this compound. We also don't start people with temporal lobe symptoms (anger, epilepsy, memory problems, hallucinations, and so on) on St. John's wort without first stabilizing the temporal lobes with anticonvulsant medication. An important note is that St. John's wort has been found to decrease the effectiveness of other drugs, including birth control pills.

5-HTP

L-tryptophan and 5-HTP are amino acid building blocks for serotonin, and using these supplements is another way to increase cerebral serotonin. L-tryptophan is a naturally occurring amino acid found in milk, meat, and eggs. It is very helpful for some patients in improving sleep, decreasing aggressiveness, and stabilizing mood. High doses of L-tryptophan in turkey are often cited as the reason we get sleepy after the Thanksgiving meal. L-tryptophan was taken off the market a number of years ago because one contaminated batch, from one manufacturer, caused a rare blood disease and a number of deaths. L-tryptophan itself actually had nothing to do with these deaths. L-tryptophan was recently reapproved by the Food and Drug Administration and is now available by prescription. One of the problems with dietary L-tryptophan is that a significant portion of it does not enter the brain but is used to make proteins and vitamin B3. This necessitates taking large amounts of tryptophan. Recommended dosage is 1,000 to 3,000 mg taken at bedtime.

5-HTP is a step closer in the serotonin-production pathway. It is also more widely available than L-tryptophan and is more easily taken up in the brain. Seventy percent is taken up into the brain, as opposed to only three percent of L-tryptophan, and 5-HTP is about five to ten times more power-ful than L-tryptophan. A number of double-blind studies have shown 5-HTP to be an effective antidepressant medication that is relatively free of the side effects caused by conventional medications. Decreased serotonin levels in the brain have been correlated with depression, aggressive feelings, and violence. 5-HTP boosts serotonin levels in the brain and helps to calm anterior cingulate gyrus hyperactivity. This is analogous to greasing (in-creasing serotonin to) the brain's gear shifter (the anterior cingulate gyrus) so that attention, focus, and concentration can be locked into place and yet also smoothly and efficiently shift onto the next item when necessary. Adults should take 5-HTP in doses of 50 to 100 mg two or three times daily with or without food, and children should take half the adult dose. Many alternative medicine doctors believe patients who are taking 5-HTP should also take 50 mg of vitamin B6 once daily because this vitamin is essential for convert-ing amino acids into serotonin. The most common side effect of 5-HTP is an upset stomach, although this is usually a mild complaint. Upset stomach can be improved by starting 5-HTP slowly and increasing the dose as you get used to the supplement and by taking it with food. Because 5-HTP increases serotonin, you should not take other medications that also increase sero-tonin, such as St. John's wort, L-tryptophan, or a prescribed antidepressant, unless you are closely supervised by your physician.

INOSITOL

Inositol is a natural biochemical found normally in the human brain. Some scientists think it is a member of the B vitamin family. It is reported to help neurons more efficiently use the neurotransmitter serotonin. In a well-designed study of thirteen patients who suffered from obsessive-compulsive disorder, 18 g of inositol compared to a placebo significantly reduced symp-toms. Spinal fluid inositol has been reported to be low in depression. An-other well-designed study of 12 g of inositol in twenty-eight depressed patients showed impressive improvement when compared to sugar pills. Since many antidepressants are effective in patients with panic disorder, twenty-one patients with this severe anxiety disorder were given 12 g of in-ositol per day for four weeks. Compared to a placebo, inositol was more ef-fective, with minimal side effects. Studies on inositol were not effective for all conditions. For example, it did not help schizophrenia, ADD, or Alzheimer's disease. By its actions and the conditions it helps, inositol seems to act like mild Prozac but with fewer of the side effects. Think of trying it if you are a worrier, have trouble letting go of negative thoughts, tend to be rigid or inflexible, or hold grudges. The dose is up to 18 g a day.

VALERIAN

Many patients find valerian to be remarkably helpful as a sleeping aid. Valerian is a well-recognized herb with antianxiety properties that is used as a mild tranquilizer, sedative, and muscle relaxant. About 150 species of valerian are widely distributed in temperate regions of the world. The active ingredient occurs in a foul-smelling oil produced in the root of the plant. The Roman physician Galen wrote about the virtues of valerian; it has been associated with the term *All Heal* in medical literature of the Middle Ages; and it is also used in Chinese and Indian medicine. It was used in the United States prior to the development of modern pharmaceuticals. This centuries-old treatment for insomnia has also been helpful for symptoms of nervousness, stress, increased emotional reactivity, pain, and agitation; it can help decrease seizure frequency for epileptic patients. Valerian appears to work by enhancing the activity of the calming neurotransmitter GABA. Studies have shown valerian to be helpful for many types of anxiety disorders and for people with performance anxiety and those who get stressed in daily situations like traffic. Valerian is available in capsules, tablets, liquids, tinctures, extracts, and teas. Most extracts are standardized to 0.8 percent valeric acids. Unlike prescription tranquilizers, valerian has a much lower potential for addiction and has been used to help people who are trying to decrease their use of prescription tranquilizers or sleeping pills. (Anyone using prescription sleeping pills or tranquilizers should decrease or stop their use only under the supervision of a physician.) Sometimes valerian can cause nervousness or drowsiness, so make sure you know how your body reacts to it before you drive or do other activities that require sustained attention. Do not take valerian with alcohol, barbiturates, or benzodiazepines. Valerian is not recommended for use during pregnancy or breastfeeding. The recommended dose of valerian is 150 to 450 mg in capsules or teas.

GETTING MORE HELP

KNOWING WHEN AND HOW TO DO IT

Even after doing all of the brain-healthy strategies in this book, some people will still need to seek professional help. Some will need psychotherapy; some will need medication; others will need more directed guidance with supplements or other alternative treatments. This chapter will help you decide if and when you need to seek professional help. In lecturing around the world, I am frequently asked: when is it time to see a professional about my brain? What should I do when a loved one is in denial about needing help? How do I go about finding a competent professional? In this chapter I will answer these questions as well as give a brief overview of several brain problems that interfere with daily living.

WHEN IS IT TIME TO SEE A PROFESSIONAL ABOUT MY BRAIN?

This question is relatively easy to answer. People should seek professional help for themselves or a family member when their behaviors, feelings, thoughts, or memories (all brain functions) interfere with their ability to reach their potential in their relationships, at work, or at school. If you are experiencing persistent relationship struggles (parent-child, sibling, friends, romantic), it's time to get help. If you have ongoing school or work problems related to your memory, moods, actions, or thoughts, it is time to get professional help. If your impulsive behavior, poor choices, or anxiety are causing consistent monetary problems, it's time to get help. Many people think they cannot afford to get professional help. I think it is usually much more costly to live with brain problems than it is to get appropriate help.

Pride and denial can get in the way of seeking proper help. People want to be strong and rely on themselves, but I am constantly reminded of the strength it takes to make the decision to get help. Also, getting help should be looked at as a way to get your brain operating at its full capacity.

Marian, whom I discussed in the Introduction, came to see me for mood swings. Even though she was very competent, her behavior at work often caused problems with her co-workers. When her boss suggested she see me, she resisted. There was nothing wrong with her, she thought—it was everyone else. One day after exploding at a co-worker, she realized it was, at least partly, her fault and agreed to come for help. She resisted because she did not want to be seen as weak or defective. The brain SPECT scan helped her to see that her brain needed to be balanced. With the appropriate help, she got better and didn't have to suffer from mood swings. She and her co-workers all suffered less stress as a result of her better-balanced brain.

WHAT SHOULD I DO WHEN A LOVED ONE IS IN DENIAL ABOUT NEEDING HELP?

Unfortunately, the stigma associated with "psychiatric illness" prevents many people from getting help. People do not want to be seen as crazy, stupid, or defective, and they do not seek help until they (or their loved one) can no longer tolerate the pain (at work, in their relationships, or within themselves). Most people do not see psychiatric problems as brain problems but rather as weak character problems. Men are especially affected by denial.

Many men, when faced with obvious troubles in their marriages, with their children, or even in themselves, are often unable to really see problems. Their lack of awareness and strong tendency toward denial prevent them from seeking help until more damage than necessary has been done. Many men have to be threatened with divorce before they seek help. Some people may say it is unfair to pick on men, and indeed some men see problems long before some women. Overall, however, mothers see problems in children before fathers and are more willing to seek help, and many more wives call for marital counseling than do husbands. What is it in our society that causes men to overlook obvious problems, or to deny problems until it is too late to deal with them effectively or until more damage is done than necessary?

Some of the answers may be found in how we raise boys, in the societal expectations we place on men, in the overwhelming pace of many men's daily lives, and in the brain.

Boys most often engage in active play (sports, war games, video games, and the like) that involve little dialogue or discussion. The games often involve dominance and submissiveness, emphasize winning and losing, and require little interpersonal communication. Force, strength, or skill handles problems. Girls, on the other hand, often engage in more interpersonal or communicative types of play, such as dolls and storytelling. Fathers often take their sons out to throw a ball around or shoot hoops rather than to go for a walk and talk.

Many men retain childhood notions of competition and the idea that one must be better than others to be any good at all. To admit to a problem is to be less than other men. As a result, many men wait to seek help until their problem has become obvious to the whole world. Other men feel responsible for all that happens in their families, so admitting to a problem is the same as admitting that they have in some way failed.

Clearly, the pace of life prevents many people, particularly men, from taking the time to look clearly at the important people in their lives and their relationships with them. When counselors spend time with fathers and husbands and help them slow down enough to see what is really important to them, more often than not they begin to see the problems and work toward more helpful solutions. The issue is generally not one of being uncaring or uninterested but of failing to see what is there. Men are wired differently from women. Men tend to be more left-brained, which gives them better access to logical, detail-oriented thought patterns. Women tend to have greater access to both sides of their brains, with the right side being involved in understanding the gestalt or big picture of a situation. The right side of the brain also seems to be involved in being able to admit to a problem. Many men just don't see problems associated with anxiety or depression, even though the symptoms may be very clear to others.

Here are several suggestions to help someone who is unaware of a problem or unwilling to get the help they need. Try the straightforward approach first (but with a new brain twist). Clearly tell the person what behaviors concern you, and explain to them that the problems may be due to underlying brain patterns that can be easily tuned up. Tell them help may be available—help not to cure a defect but rather to optimize how their brain functions. Tell them you know they are trying to do their best, but their behavior, thoughts, or feelings may be getting in the way of their success (at work, in relationships, or within themselves). Emphasize better function, not defect.

Give them information. Books, videos, and articles on the subjects you are concerned about can be of tremendous help. Many people come to the Amen Clinics because they read a book, saw a video, or read an article. Good information can be very persuasive, especially if it is presented in a positive, life-enhancing way.

If the person remains resistant to help, even after you have been straightforward and given them good information, plant seeds. Plant ideas about getting help, then water them regularly. Drop an idea, article, or other source of information about the topic from time to time. If you talk too much about getting help, people become resentful and will refuse to get help to spite you, especially the overfocused types. Be careful not to go overboard.

Protect your relationship with the other person. People are more receptive to people they trust than to people who nag and belittle them. Work on gaining the person's trust over the long run. It will make them more receptive to your suggestions. Do not make getting help the only thing you talk about. Make sure you are interested in their whole lives, not just in their potential medical appointments.

Give them new hope. Many people with these problems have tried to get help, and it did not work or even made them worse. Educate them on new brain technology that helps professionals be more focused and more effective in their treatment efforts.

There comes a time when you have to say, enough is enough. If, over time, the other person refuses to get help, and his or her behavior has a negative impact on your life, you may have to separate yourself. Staying in a toxic relationship is harmful to your health, and it often enables the other person to remain sick as well. Actually, I have seen that the threat or act of leaving motivates people to change, whether it is about drinking, drug use, or treating ADD. Threatening to leave is not the first approach I would take, but after time it may be the best approach. Realize that you cannot force a person into treatment unless they are dangerous to themselves, dangerous to others, or unable to care for themselves. You can only do what you can do. Fortunately, we can do a lot more today than we could even ten years ago.

FINDING A COMPETENT PROFESSIONAL WHO USES
THIS NEW BRAIN SCIENCE THINKING

The Amen Clinics get many calls, faxes, and e-mails each week from people all over the world looking for competent professionals in their area who think in similar ways to the principles outlined in this book. Because this approach is on the edge of what is new in brain science, other professionals who know and practice this information may be hard to find. But finding the right professional for evaluation and treatment is critical to the healing process. The right professional can have a very positive impact on your life; the wrong professional can make things worse.

There are a number of steps you can take to find the best person to assist you. Get the best person you can find. Saving money up front by choosing someone less expensive but also less able may cost you in the long run. The right help is not only cost effective but saves unnecessary pain and suffering, so don't rely on a person simply because they are on your managed care plan. That person may or may not be a good fit for you. Search for the best. If he or she is on your insurance plan, great, but don't let that be the primary criterion. Once you get the names of competent professionals, check their credentials. Very few patients ever check a professional's background. Board certification is a positive credential. To become board certified, physicians must pass additional written and verbal tests. They have to discipline themselves to gain the levels of skill and knowledge that are acceptable to their colleagues. Don't give too much weight to the medical school or graduate school the professional attended. I have worked with doctors who went to Yale and Harvard who did not have a clue as to how to appropriately treat patients, while other doctors from less prestigious schools were outstanding, forward thinking, and caring. Set up an interview with the professional to see whether you want to work with him or her. Generally you have to pay for their time, but it is worth spending the money to get to know the people you will rely on for help.

Many professionals write articles or books or speak at meetings or local groups. Read the professional's work or hear him or her speak, if possible. By doing so you may be able to get a feel for the kind of person they are and their ability to help you. Look for a person who is open-minded, up-to-date, and willing to try new things. Look for a person who treats you with respect, who listens to your questions and responds to your needs. Look for a relationship that is collaborative and respectful. I know it is hard to find a professional who meets all of these criteria who also has the right training in brain physiology, but these people can be found. Be persistent. The caregiver is essential to healing.

A QUICK VIEW OF COMMON BRAIN PROBLEMS NEEDING HELP

I once got a phone call from a very close friend whom I hadn't heard from in years. He sounded different. When we lived close together, he had been energetic, positive, outgoing, funny, and fascinated by the world around him. As I listened to him that day on the phone, however, his voice was flat, and his thoughts were very negative. He told me his life had no meaning and that he would much rather "see heaven" than struggle through any more days. My friend was sleeping a lot, had problems concentrating, and had even lost interest in sex, which was a real change for him. He was suffering from a clinical depression. He was the last person in the world with whom I expected to be having that kind of conversation. But brain illnesses affecting emotions, behaviors, and learning are very common. A study sponsored by the National Institute of Mental Health reported that 49 percent of the population will suffer from a mental illness (really a brain illness) during some point in their life. Mood problems, anxiety disorders, alcohol or drug abuse, and attention deficit disorders are the most common problems. Mental illnesses strike the rich and the poor, the successful and the not so successful. They devastate individuals and families, and they often go untreated because of the stigma our society attaches to them.

My friend had postponed calling me for over nine months. Not until his wife threatened to divorce him did he call me. Many uninformed people have the erroneous idea that people with emotional illnesses are strange, scary, or way out there. True, some people with mental illnesses have delusions or are violent, but the vast majority of those who suffer from anxiety, depression, or drug use are more like you and me than they are different; left untreated, these problems seriously undermine people's ability to be their best self.

What follows is a brief synopsis of mood disorders, anxiety problems, substance abuse, and attention deficit disorder. Whenever I evaluate a new patient, I take a bio/psycho/social approach. That means I look at the biological, psychological, and social causes that may be underlying the problem. In addition, I also look at brain scans to subtype brain illnesses. For example, I have seen seven different types of anxiety and depression and six different types of ADD. We work to target treatment to enhance the underlying brain systems that may be involved in the problem. See my books *Healing Anxiety and Depression* and *Healing ADD* for a full discussion of subtyping these illnesses.

MOOD DISORDERS

DEPRESSION

Janet, a forty-two-year-old lawyer, wife, and mother of three, was referred to me because she was tired all the time. Her family physician ruled out the physical causes of fatigue and thought she was overstressed. Additionally, she had trouble concentrating at work and experienced difficulty sleeping. Her sex drive was gone, her appetite was poor, and she had no interest in doing things with her family. She would start to cry for no apparent reason, and she even began to entertain desperate suicidal thoughts. Janet had a serious depressive illness.

Depression is a very common mental illness. Studies reveal that at any point in time, 3 to 6 percent of the population has a significant depression. Only 20 to 25 percent of these people ever seek help. This is unfortunate because depression is a very treatable problem.

The following is a list of symptoms commonly associated with depression:

- sad, blue, or gloomy mood
- low energy, frequent fatigue
- lack of ability to feel pleasure in usually pleasurable activities
- irritability
- poor concentration, distractibility, poor memory
- suicidal thoughts, feelings of meaninglessness
- feelings of hopelessness, helplessness, guilt, and worthlessness
- changes in sleep, either poor sleep with frequent awakenings or increased sleep
- changes in appetite, either markedly decreased or increased
- social withdrawal
- low self-esteem

Here is an example of the bio/psycho/social approach to understanding depression. There are several important biological factors to look for in depression.

- Family history. Depression often has a genetic link, and it often runs in families where there has been alcohol abuse.

- Medical evaluation. A number of illnesses can cause depression, including thyroid disease, infectious illnesses, cancer, and certain forms of anemia. A heart attack, stroke, or brain trauma can also leave a person vulnerable to depression.
- Dramatic hormonal shifts (postpartum or menopausal). Such shifts often precipitate problems with depression.
- Medications. Certain medications can cause depression, most notably birth control pills, certain blood pressure or cardiac medications, steroids, and chronic pain control medicines.
- Alcohol and drug abuse history. Chronic alcohol or marijuana use often causes depression, while amphetamine or cocaine withdrawal is often accompanied by serious suicidal thoughts.

The psychological factors to look for in depression include:

- A major loss. The death of a loved one, the breakup of a romantic relationship, the loss of a job, of self-esteem, status, health, or purpose—all can cause depression.
- Multiple childhood traumas, such as physical or sexual abuse. These too can cause depression.
- Negative thinking. Negative thoughts erode self-esteem and drive mood down.
- Learned helplessness, the belief that no matter what you do things won't change. This comes from being exposed to environments where you are continually frustrated in reaching your goals.

The social factors or current life stresses to evaluate in depression include:

- Marital problems
- Family dysfunction
- Financial difficulties
- Work-related problems

In Janet's case, her physical examination was normal, but her father had had periods of depression, and she had an uncle who killed himself. Psychologically, she had a very critical mother, and subsequently she was extremely self-critical. Socially, her marriage had been difficult for the past several years, and she was often fighting with her teenage son.

The best results in treating any emotional illness occur with a bio/psy-cho/social approach. Janet was placed on antidepressant medication and learned to be significantly less critical of herself. We also spent time working on her marriage and her relationship with her teenage son. In ten weeks she felt more energetic and was able to concentrate. Her mood was good. She slept well and her appetite returned. She also got along better at home with her husband and son.

Depression is a very treatable illness. Early detection and treatment from a bio/psycho/social perspective is important to a full and complete recovery. From a biological standpoint, we think of medication or supplements and proper diet and exercise. Exercise has been found in some studies to be as effective as medication, but cheaper and with fewer side effects. (Most of the side effects of exercise are positive.) Psychotherapy has also been found to be helpful in treating depression. The two best-studied forms of psychotherapy for depression are cognitive therapy, which teaches patients to counteract the negative thoughts that invariably surface with depression, and interpersonal psychotherapy, which teaches patients to have more effective relationships.

BIPOLAR DISORDER

Another type of mood disorder is bipolar disorder, in which people cycle between two poles. Periods of depression may alternate with periods of high, manic, irritable, or elated moods. Mania is categorized as a state distinct from one's normal self, where one has greater energy, racing thoughts, more impulsivity, a decreased need for sleep, and a sense of grandiosity. It is often associated with periods of hypersexuality, hyperreligiosity, and spending sprees. Sometimes it is also associated with hallucinations or delusions. In treating the depressive part of the cycle, both pharmaceutical and supplement antidepressants have been known to stimulate manic episodes. It is important to vigorously treat this disorder, as it has been associated with marital problems, substance abuse, and suicide.

Here is a list of symptoms often associated with bipolar disorder.

- Periods of abnormally elevated, depressed, or anxious mood
- Periods of decreased need for sleep, feeling energetic on dramatically less sleep than usual
- Periods of grandiose notions, ideas, or plans
- Periods of increased talking or pressured speech

- Periods of too many thoughts racing through the mind
- Periods of markedly increased energy
- Periods of poor judgment that leads to risk-taking behavior (separate from usual behavior)
- Periods of inappropriate social behavior
- Periods of irritability or aggression
- Periods of delusional or psychotic thinking

The classic form of this disorder is known as Bipolar I, which used to be called manic-depressive illness. In recent years, a milder form of the disorder called Bipolar II has been associated with depressive episodes and milder "hypomanic" issues.

The treatment for bipolar disorder, both I and II, is usually medication, such as lithium or anticonvulsants such as Depakote. In recent years literature suggests that high doses of omega-3 fatty acids, found in fish and flaxseed oils, can also be helpful.

ANXIETY DISORDERS

There are four common types of anxiety disorders that can affect people in a negative way: panic disorder, agoraphobia, obsessive-compulsive disorder, and post-traumatic stress disorder. I'll briefly discuss each of these and their treatments.

PANIC DISORDER

All of a sudden your heart starts to pound. You get this feeling of incredible dread. Your breathing rate goes faster. You start to sweat. Your muscles get tight, and your hands feel like ice. Your mind starts to race about every terrible thing that could possibly happen, and you feel as though you're going to lose your mind if you don't get out of the current situation. You've just had a panic attack. Panic attacks are one of the most common brain disorders. It is estimated that 6 to 7 percent of adults will at some point in their lives suffer from recurrent panic attacks. They often begin in late adolescence or early adulthood but may spontaneously occur later in life. If a person has three attacks in a three-week period, doctors make a diagnosis of a panic disorder.

In a typical panic attack, a person has at least four of the following twelve symptoms: shortness of breath, heart pounding, chest pain, choking or smothering feelings, dizziness, tingling of hands or feet, feeling unreal, hot or cold flashes, sweating, faintness, trembling or shaking, and a fear of dying or going crazy. When a panic attack first starts, many people end up in the emergency room because they think they're having a heart attack. Some people even end up being admitted to the hospital.

Anticipation anxiety is one of the most difficult symptoms for people who have a panic disorder. These people are often extremely skilled at predicting the worst in a situation. In fact, it is often the anticipation of a bad event that brings on a panic attack. For example, you are in the grocery store and worry that you're going to have an anxiety attack and pass out on the floor. Then, you predict, everyone in the store will look at you and laugh. Pretty quickly the symptoms begin. Sometimes a panic disorder can become so severe that a person begins to avoid almost any situation outside of their house, a condition called agoraphobia.

Panic attacks can occur for a variety of different reasons. Sometimes they are caused by a medical illness, such as hyperthyroidism, which is why it's always important to have a physical examination and screening blood work. Sometimes they can be brought on by excessive caffeine intake or alcohol withdrawal. Hormonal changes also seem to play a role. Panic attacks in women are seen more frequently at the end of their menstrual cycle, after having a baby, and during menopause. Traumatic events from the past that somehow get unconsciously triggered can also precipitate a series of attacks. Commonly there is a family history of panic attacks, alcohol abuse, or other mental illnesses.

On SPECT scans we often see hyperactivity in the basal ganglia or sometimes in the temporal lobe. Psychotherapy is my preferred treatment for this disorder, and in some studies it has been shown to calm basal ganglia activity. Sometimes supplements or medications can be helpful. Unfortunately the most helpful medications are also addictive, so care is needed.

AGORAPHOBIA

The name *agoraphobia* comes from a Greek word that means "fear of the marketplace." In behavioral terms it means fear of being alone in public places. The person's underlying worry is that they will lose control or become incapacitated and no one will be there to help. People afflicted with this phobia avoid being in crowds, in stores, or on busy streets. They're often afraid of being in tunnels, on bridges, in elevators, or on public transportation. They usually insist that a family member or a friend accompany them when they leave home. If the fear establishes a foothold in the person, it may affect his or her whole life. Normal activities become increasingly restricted as the fears and avoidance behaviors dominate their life.

Agoraphobic symptoms often begin in the late teen years or early twenties, but I've seen them start in people in their fifties and sixties. Often, without knowing what is wrong, agoraphobic people will try to medicate themselves with excessive amounts of alcohol or drugs. This illness occurs more frequently in women, and many of those who have it experienced significant separation anxiety as children. Additionally, there may be a history of excessive anxiety, panic attacks, depression, or alcohol abuse in relatives.

Agoraphobia often evolves out of panic attacks that seem to occur "out of the blue," for no apparent reason. These attacks are so frightening that the person begins to avoid any situation that may be in any way associated with the fear. I think these initial panic attacks are often triggered by an unconscious memory of an event or by an anxiety from the past. For example, I once treated a patient who had been raped as a teenager in a park late at night. When she was twenty-eight, she had her first panic attack while walking late at night in a park with her husband. She associated the park setting late at night with being raped, which triggered the panic attack.

Agoraphobia is a very frightening illness both to the patient and to his or her family. With effective, early intervention, however, there is significant hope for recovery. The scan findings and treatment are similar to those for people with panic disorder. The one difference is that people with agoraphobia often have increased anterior cingulate gyrus activity and get stuck in their fear of having more panic attacks. Getting stuck in the fear often prevents them from leaving home. Using medications, such as Prozac and Lexapro, or supplements, such as 5-HTP and St. John's wort, to increase serotonin and calm this part of the brain is often helpful.

OBSESSIVE-COMPULSIVE DISORDER

The hallmarks of obsessive-compulsive disorder (OCD) are recurrent thoughts that seem outside a person's control, or compulsive behaviors that a person knows make no sense but that he or she feels compelled to do anyway. The obsessive thoughts may involve violence (such as killing one's child), contamination (such as becoming infected by shaking hands), or doubt (such as the worry of having hurt someone in a traffic accident, even though no such accident occurred). Many efforts are made to suppress or resist these thoughts, but the more a person tries to control them, the more powerful they can become.

The most common compulsions involve hand-washing, counting, checking, and touching. These behaviors are often performed according to certain rules in a very strict or rigid manner. For example, people with a counting compulsion may feel the need to count every crack on the pavement on their way to work or school. What would be a five-minute walk for most people could turn into a three- or four-hour trip for the person with OCD. They have an urgent sense of "I have to do it" inside. A part of the individual generally recognizes the senselessness of the behavior and doesn't get pleasure from carrying it out, although doing it often provides a release of tension. Over the years I've treated many people with OCD, the youngest of whom was five years old. He had a checking compulsion and had to check the house locks at night as many as twenty to thirty times before he could fall asleep. The oldest person I treated with this disorder was eighty-three. She had obsessive sexual thoughts that made her feel dirty inside. It got to the point where she would lock all her doors, draw all the window shades, turn off the lights, take the phone off the hook, and sit in the middle of a dark room trying to catch the abhorrent sexual thoughts as they came into her mind.

On SPECT studies of people with OCD, we often see excessive activity in the basal ganglia and anterior cingulate gyrus. Behavior therapy can be helpful and has been shown to improve brain function. Using medications, such as Prozac and Lexapro, or supplements, such as 5-HTP and St. John's wort, to increase serotonin and calm these parts of the brain is often helpful.

POST-TRAUMATIC STRESS DISORDER

Joanne, a thirty-four-year-old travel agent, was held up in her office at gunpoint by two men. Four or five times during the robbery, one of the men held a gun to her head and said he was going to kill her. She graphically imagined her brain being splattered with blood against the wall. Near the end of this fifteen-minute ordeal they made her take off all her clothes. She pictured herself being brutally raped by them. They left without touching her, locked in a closet.

Since that time her life had been thrown into turmoil. She felt tense and was plagued with flashbacks and nightmares of the robbery. Her stomach was in knots, and she had a constant headache. Whenever she went out, she felt panicky. She was frustrated that she could not calm her body: her heart raced, she was short of breath, and her hands were constantly cold and sweaty. She hated how she felt, and she was angry about how her nice life had turned into a nightmare. What was most upsetting to her were the ways the robbery affected her marriage and her child. Her baby picked up the tension and was very fussy. Every time she tried to make love with her husband, she began to cry and get images of the men raping her.

Joanne had post-traumatic stress disorder (PTSD), a brain reaction to a severe traumatic event such as a robbery, rape, car accident, earthquake, tornado, or even a volcanic eruption. Her symptoms were classic for PTSD, especially the flashbacks and nightmares of the event.

Perhaps the worst symptoms, however, came from the horrible thoughts about what had never happened, such as seeing her brain splattered against the wall and being raped. These thoughts were registered in her subconscious as fact, and until she entered treatment she was not able to recognize how much damage they had been doing to her. For example, when she imagined that she was being raped, a part of her began to believe that she actually was raped. The first time she had her period after the robbery, she began to cry because she was relieved she was not pregnant by the robbers, even though they never touched her. A part of her even believed she was dead because she had so vividly pictured her own death. A significant portion of her treatment was geared to counteract these erroneous subconscious conclusions.

Without treatment, PTSD can literally ruin a person's life. The most effective treatment is usually psychotherapy. One type of psychotherapy that I think works especially well for PTSD is Eye Movement Desensitization and Reprocessing (EMDR). You can learn more about this technique in my book *Healing Anxiety and Depression* or by visiting www.emdria.org. Depending on the severity of PTSD, certain types of medications and supplements can also be helpful.

DRUG AND ALCOHOL ABUSE

Many people use alcohol or drugs to medicate underlying brain systems that are misfiring. Downers, such as alcohol, marijuana, sedatives, and pain-killers, are used to calm hyperactive brain systems; uppers, such as cocaine and methamphetamine, are used to stimulate underactive areas of the brain. The problem is that most of these substances are addictive and cause brain damage. Sometimes the damage is permanent. In addition, substance abuse has a serious negative impact on relationships, work, and health. In relationships, many people complain that their partner who is abusing these substances is emotional, erratic, selfish, and unpredictable. Alcohol and drug abuse are common causes of relationship breakups. The list of health problems caused by alcohol and drugs fills volumes of books. The most common workplace problems include erratic job performance, absenteeism, tardiness, work accidents, and decreased job performance. Denial is frequently strong in substance abusers. The person with the problem is usually the last one to recognize that a problem is present. Alcohol- and drug-related problems are similar in many ways. I have chosen to lump these two groups together for simplicity.

Note: *Alcohol* means any beverage or medication that contains any alcohol, from beer or wine to hard liquor, and even some cough preparations. *Drug* means any mind-altering substance that produces a stimulant, depressant, or euphoric effect—amphetamines, barbiturates, marijuana, cocaine, heroin, PCP, and so on.

Go through the following list of symptoms of excessive alcohol or drug use, and check off those that apply to you. This will give you an idea if this area is a problem for you or someone you know.

1. Increasing consumption of alcohol or drugs, whether on a regular or a sporadic basis, with frequent and perhaps unintended episodes of intoxication
2. Use of drugs or alcohol as a means of handling problems
3. Obvious preoccupation with alcohol or drugs and the expressed need to have them
4. Gulping of drinks or using large quantities of drugs
5. Need for increasing quantities of alcohol or the drug to obtain the same "buzz"
6. Tendency to make alibis and weak excuses for drinking or drug use
7. Need to have others cover for you, either at work or at home
8. Refusal to concede what is obviously excessive consumption and expressing annoyance when the subject is mentioned
9. Frequent absenteeism from the job, especially if it occurs in a pattern, such as following weekends and holidays (Monday morning "flu")

10. Repeated changes in jobs, particularly to successively lower levels, or employment in a capacity beneath one's ability, education, and background

11. Shabby appearance, poor hygiene, and behavior and social adjustment inconsistent with previous levels or expectations

12. Persistent vague body complaints without apparent cause, particularly trouble sleeping, abdominal problems, headaches, or loss of appetite

13. Multiple contacts with the health care system

14. Persistent marital problems; perhaps multiple marriages

15. History of arrests for intoxicated driving or disorderly conduct

16. Unusual anxiety or obvious moodiness

17. Withdrawal symptoms on stopping (tremors, feeling extremely anxious, craving drugs or alcohol, vomiting, and so on); an alcoholic or drug abuser has usually tried to stop many times but is unable to withstand the symptoms of withdrawal

18. Hearing voices or seeing things that aren't there

19. Blackouts (times you cannot remember)

20. Memory impairment

21. Drinking or using drugs alone; early-morning use; secretive use

22. *Denial* in the face of an obvious problem

My favorite definition of an alcoholic or drug addict is anyone who has gotten into trouble (legal, relational, or work-related) while drinking or using the drug, then continues to use it. They did not learn from the previous experience. A rational person would realize that he or she has trouble handling the alcohol or drug and would stay away from it. Unfortunately, many people with these problems have to experience repeated failures because of the substance use and thus hit "rock bottom" before treatment is sought.

A very helpful trend in medicine over the last ten years has been to classify alcoholism and excessive drug use as illnesses instead of morally weak behavior. The American Medical Association, the World Health Organization, and many other professional groups regard these as specific disease entities.

Untreated, these diseases progress to serious physical complications that often lead to death. Here are some important facts you need to know about alcohol and drug abuse.

1. These addictions often run in families. The more relatives a person has who are alcoholics or addicts, the more likely they are or will be-

come dependent on these chemicals. A rule of thumb: one parent = 25 percent chance; two parents or one parent and one sibling = 50 percent chance; three or more family members = 75-plus percent chance.

2. Alcoholism or drug addiction shortens life expectancy by an estimated ten to fifteen years.
3. Alcoholism and drug addictions occur in about fifteen million Americans. If this problem applies to you, you are not alone.
4. There is no typical person with alcoholism or a drug addiction. These diseases affect people in all socioeconomic classes.
5. Drunken driving or driving under the influence of drugs is responsible for well over 50 percent of all highway traffic fatalities.
6. Alcoholism and drug addiction are treatable. Treatment for alcohol or drug abusers and their families is widely available today in all parts of the country.

In treating substance abuse, it is important to recognize and treat any underlying cause of the problem, such as unrecognized depression, bipolar disorder, anxiety disorders, or ADD. New medications have been developed that have been found helpful in alleviating withdrawal symptoms and decreasing cravings for the substances. Psychotherapy and support groups are often helpful as well.

ATTENTION DEFICIT DISORDER

Do you often feel restless? Have trouble concentrating? Have trouble with impulsiveness, either doing or saying things you wish you hadn't? Do you fail to finish many projects you start? Are you easily bored or quick to anger? If the answer to most of these questions is yes, you may have attention deficit disorder (ADD).

ADD is the most common brain problem in children, affecting 5 to 10 percent of them in the United States, and one of the most common problems in adults. The main symptoms of ADD are a short attention span, distractibility, disorganization, procrastination, and poor internal supervision. It is often, but not always, associated with impulsive behavior and hyperactivity or restlessness. Until recently most people thought children outgrew this disorder during their teenage years. For many, this is false. While it is true that the hyperactivity lessens over time, the other symptoms of impulsivity, distractibility, and a short attention span remain for most sufferers into adulthood. Current research shows that 60 to 80 percent of ADD children never fully outgrow this disorder. Over the years I have seen thousands of children who had ADD. When I meet with their parents and take a good family history, I find that there is about an 80 percent chance that at least one of the parents also had symptoms of ADD as a child and may, in fact, still be showing symptoms as an adult. Many of the parents were never diagnosed. Not infrequently I learn of ADD in adults when parents tell me that they tried their child's medication (not something I recommend) and found it very helpful. They report it helped them concentrate for longer periods of time and that they become more organized and less impulsive.

Common symptoms of the adult form of ADD include poor organization and planning, procrastination, trouble listening carefully to directions, and excessive traffic violations. Additionally, people with adult ADD are often late for appointments, frequently misplace things, may be quick to anger, and have poor follow-through. There may also be frequent, impulsive job changes and poor financial management. Substance abuse, especially of alcohol or amphetamines and cocaine, and low self-esteem are also common.

Many people do not recognize the seriousness of this disorder and just pass these kids and adults off as lazy, defiant, or willful. But ADD is a serious disorder. Left untreated, it affects a person's self-esteem, social relationships, and ability to learn and work. Several studies have shown that ADD children use twice as many medical services as non-ADD kids. Up to 35 percent of untreated ADD teens never finish high school, 52 percent of untreated adults abuse substances, teens and adults with ADD have more traffic accidents, and adults with ADD move four times more than others.

Many adults tell me that when they were children they were in trouble all the time and had a real sense that there was something very different about them. Even though many of the adults I treat with ADD are very bright, they are frequently frustrated by not living up to their potential.

Our research with SPECT scans makes it clear that ADD is a brain disorder, but not one simple disorder. I have described six different types of ADD. The most common feature of ADD is decreased activity in the prefrontal cortex with a concentration task. This means that the harder a person tries, the less brain activity they have to work with. Many people with ADD self-medicate with stimulants—such as caffeine, nicotine, cocaine, or methamphetamine—to increase activity in the PFC. They also tend to self-medicate with conflict-seeking behavior. If they can get someone upset, it helps to stimulate their brain. Of course, they have no idea they do this behavior. I call it unconscious, brain-driven behavior. But if you are around ADD people long enough, you will see and feel the conflict-seeking behavior.

The best treatment for ADD depends on the type of ADD a person has. See my book *Healing ADD* for a complete description of types and treatments. In general, intense exercise helps, as does a higher-protein, lower-carbohydrate diet. Sometimes medications or supplements are helpful, but they can make things worse if they are not right. When correctly targeted, ADD is a highly treatable disorder in both children and adults.

Do not let pride get in the way of getting the help you need. In order to make a good brain great, you have to admit when you need help. Remember Principle 9, we all need a little help.

FIFTEEN DAYS TO A
BETTER BRAIN

Give your brain one hour a day for fifteen days, and you will be on your way to making your good brain great. Of course, you will need to keep up the program over time, but you will notice a dramatic difference in just two weeks and one day, and you'll be on the road to the best brain possible. Here are six steps to putting the program together.

STEP ONE

Buy or make a journal.

STEP TWO

On page one write out your "One-Page Miracle" (see Chapter 16). Spend a good part of day one completing it. It will be your road map to success.

STEP THREE

On the next page, compose a poem or letter to your brain. As silly as it sounds, it is important to do some bonding exercises with your brain. Love and emotion help motivate us into action. Here's an example—I call it "A Love Letter to My Brain."

A LOVE LETTER TO MY BRAIN

To My Beloved Brain:

You are involved in everything I do. When you work right, I work right; when you are troubled or in a bad way, I tend struggle with life. You are extraordinary, wondrous, complicated, and sometimes hard to understand. You are also very fragile, soft, and in need of protection from harm. Since you are 85 percent water, I know you need lots of fresh water every day. You are multitalented . . . certain parts of you do certain things really well and help me in many areas of life. I know that sometimes you also can have trouble. I am sorry when you hurt or don't function at your best. We need to become more intimate and get to know each other better. If you need help, I am here for you. If needed, we will look under the hood. I will not allow people to guess at what you need without looking at you. Using emotion (from the limbic system) and directed effort (from the prefrontal cortex) we can change; we can make each other better and happier, starting today. I will not expect you to be perfect, because we all need a little help.

STEP FOUR

Next, write down the promises that you are willing to make to your brain. Here are some examples.

In a sincere effort to keep you healthy so that we can have a long, happy, productive life together, I am willing to make you the following promises. I promise that I will:

- Think about you every day, so you can think properly
- Care for you, so you will allow me to take good care of myself and those I love
- Accept the fact their neither you nor I are perfect, but we can be better
- Protect you from injury, toxins, and too much stress
- Give you enough sleep
- Feed you nutritious food, but not too much
- Teach you new things so you continue to be excellent at learning
- Exercise our heart and body to keep great blood supply flowing to you
- Keep you coordinated so we can think and act faster
- Keep you physically and emotionally connected to others
- Play beautiful music for you so that your firing patterns will stay healthy

- Actively seek to prevent diseases of aging so we can stay young together
- Give you the supplements you need to help keep you healthy
- Get you help when needed

STEP FIVE

Next, label the journal pages one to ten. On each page write all the following headings:

- Exercise. Write the time and level of exercise you did that day. Strive toward at least thirty minutes a day where you get your heart rate up above normal.
- Supplements. Write down each supplement that you take each day; I recommend the following cocktail for most adults (see Chapter 20 for more details):
  - Acetyl-L-carnitine—500 mg once a day
  - Alpha-lipoic acid—100 mg once a day
  - Fish oil—1,000 mg twice a day
  - Phosphatidylserine—100 mg twice a day
  - Super multiple vitamin with high-dose B vitamins
  - Vitamin E (mixed tocopherols)—100 mg twice a day
  - Vitamin C—250 mg twice a day
- Meditation. Write down the time you spent meditating or doing relaxation exercises. Strive for twelve minutes a day for mental clarity and stress management. I recommend an active form of yoga meditation called Kriya Kirtan. It is based on the five primal sounds saa, taa, naa, maa, and aa. Repeat each sound as you consecutively touch your thumb to fingers two, three, four, and five. Repeat the sounds and fingering for two minutes out loud, two minutes whispering, four minutes silently, two minutes whispering, and two minutes out loud. It is okay to make a tape or set a quiet alarm to keep the timing accurate.
- New learning. Spend at least fifteen minutes a day learning something new, and write down what you learned in your journal.
- What I ate today. Include the food and drinks you consume each day, including snacks. For the first two weeks give a general idea of the calories you consume. If you don't know, start to measure and count. Remember, calorie restriction is a brain longevity strategy.

STEP SIX

Let's get started!!

DAY 1: FIRST THINGS FIRST

Complete your own One-Page Miracle (see Chapter 16 for directions)

- Exercise _____ (percent of targeted thirty-minute exercise accomplished)
- Supplements _____ (yes or no)
- Meditation _____ (time spent; target twelve minutes a day)
- New learning _____ (what new piece of information or new skill did you learn today?)
- What I ate today (list the food and approximate calories you ate today)
  Breakfast _____
  Snack _____
  Lunch _____
  Snack _____
  Dinner _____
  Dessert _____
  Approximate calories _____

DAY 2: A LOVE LETTER TO MY BRAIN

Write a poem or love letter to your brain.

- Exercise _____ (percent of targeted thirty-minute exercise accomplished)
- Supplements _____ (yes or no)
- Meditation _____ (time spent; target twelve minutes a day)
- New learning _____ (what new piece of information or new skill did you learn today?)
- What I ate today (list the food and approximate calories you ate today)
  Breakfast _____
  Snack _____
  Lunch _____
  Snack _____
  Dinner _____
  Dessert _____
  Approximate calories _____

DAY 3: PROMISES TO MY BRAIN

Write your promises to your brain.

- Exercise _____ (percent of targeted thirty-minute exercise accomplished)
- Supplements _____ (yes or no)
- Meditation _____ (time spent; target twelve minutes a day)
- New learning _____ (what new piece of information or new skill did you learn today?)
- What I ate today (list the food and approximate calories you ate today)
  Breakfast _____
  Snack _____
  Lunch _____
  Snack _____
  Dinner _____
  Dessert _____
  Approximate calories _____

DAY 4: WORKING THE BRAIN

New learning takes priority. What have you always wanted to study or know more about?

- Exercise _____ (percent of targeted thirty-minute exercise accomplished)
- Supplements _____ (yes or no)
- Meditation _____ (time spent; target twelve minutes a day)
- New learning _____ (what new piece of information or new skill did you learn today?)
- What I ate today (list the food and approximate calories you ate today)
  Breakfast _____
  Snack _____
  Lunch _____
  Snack _____
  Dinner _____
  Dessert _____
  Approximate calories _____

DAY 5: FEEDING THE BRAIN

Make all your food today from recipes containing brain-healthy ingredients (see Chapter 11). Here is a summary.

Protein: salmon, chicken, turkey, eggs, tofu and soy products, low-fat dairy, beans, nuts/seeds

Carbs: berries, oranges, cherries, broccoli, oats, whole wheat, wheat germ, red peppers, spinach, tomatoes, yams

Fats: avocados, olive oil, olives, nut butter

Liquids: water, green or black tea

- Exercise _____ (percent of targeted thirty-minute exercise accomplished)
- Supplements _____ (yes or no)
- Meditation _____ (time spent; target twelve minutes a day)
- New learning _____ (what new piece of information or new skill did you learn today?)
- What I ate today (list the food and approximate calories you ate today)
    Breakfast _____
    Snack _____
    Lunch _____
    Snack _____
    Dinner _____
    Dessert _____
    Approximate calories _____

DAY 6: GREAT MUSIC DAY

Incorporate new music into your day. Try Mozart or some other classical piece if that kind of music is new for you.

- Exercise _____ (percent of targeted thirty-minute exercise accomplished)
- Supplements _____ (yes or no)
- Meditation _____ (time spent; target twelve minutes a day)
- New learning _____ (what new piece of information or new skill did you learn today?)
- What I ate today (list the food and approximate calories you ate today)
  Breakfast _____
  Snack _____
  Lunch _____
  Snack _____
  Dinner _____
  Dessert _____
  Approximate calories _____

DAY 7: A CALMING DAY

Put aside the time to meditate twice today.

- Exercise _____ (percent of targeted thirty-minute exercise accomplished)
- Supplements _____ (yes or no)
- Meditation _____ (time spent; target twelve minutes a day)
- New learning _____ (what new piece of information or new skill did you learn today?)
- What I ate today (list the food and approximate calories you ate today)
  Breakfast _____
  Snack _____
  Lunch _____
  Snack _____
  Dinner _____
  Dessert _____
  Approximate calories _____

DAY 8: A NEW COORDINATION EXERCISE

Try a new sport today—maybe even table tennis, but take lessons so it is more than basement Ping-Pong.

- Exercise _____ (percent of targeted thirty-minute exercise accomplished)
- Supplements _____ (yes or no)
- Meditation _____ (time spent; target twelve minutes a day)
- New learning _____ (what new piece of information or new skill did you learn today?)
- What I ate today (list the food and approximate calories you ate today)
  Breakfast _____
  Snack _____
  Lunch _____
  Snack _____
  Dinner _____
  Dessert _____
  Approximate calories _____

DAY 9: GRATEFUL DAY

List ten things you are grateful for today, and focus on them throughout the day.

- Exercise _____ (percent of targeted thirty-minute exercise accomplished)
- Supplements _____ (yes or no)
- Meditation _____ (time spent; target twelve minutes a day)
- New learning _____ (what new piece of information or new skill did you learn today?)
- What I ate today (list the food and approximate calories you ate today)
  Breakfast _____
  Snack _____
  Lunch _____
  Snack _____
  Dinner _____
  Dessert _____
  Approximate calories _____

DAY 10: EXTRA SLEEP

Get an hour more sleep than you usually do—stop the sleep-deprived life you have been living, at least for a day.

- Exercise _____ (percent of targeted thirty-minute exercise accomplished)
- Supplements _____ (yes or no)
- Meditation _____ (time spent; target twelve minutes a day)
- New learning _____ (what new piece of information or new skill did you learn today?)
- What I ate today (list the food and approximate calories you ate today)
    Breakfast _____
    Snack _____
    Lunch _____
    Snack _____
    Dinner _____
    Dessert _____
    Approximate calories _____

DAY 11: NO TV, VIDEO GAME, OR COMPUTER DAY

TV, video games, and excessive computer play are not great for the brain. Take a day off to unplug your brain and see how it feels. Odds are you will figure out something more creative to do with your brain.

- Exercise _____ (percent of targeted thirty-minute exercise accomplished)
- Supplements _____ (yes or no)
- Meditation _____ (time spent; target twelve minutes a day)
- New learning _____ (what new piece of information or new skill did you learn today?)
- What I ate today (list the food and approximate calories you ate today)
    Breakfast _____
    Snack _____
    Lunch _____
    Snack _____
    Dinner _____
    Dessert _____
    Approximate calories _____

DAY 12: PHYSICAL AFFECTION DAY

If you are in a committed relationship, make love twice today. Feel the oxytocin bathe your brain in bonding chemicals. If not, spend time with people you love, and make sure to hug each other and smile.

- Exercise _____ (percent of targeted thirty-minute exercise accomplished)
- Supplements _____ (yes or no)
- Meditation _____ (time spent; target twelve minutes a day)
- New learning _____ (what new piece of information or new skill did you learn today?)
- What I ate today (list the food and approximate calories you ate today)
  Breakfast _____
  Snack _____
  Lunch _____
  Snack _____
  Dinner _____
  Dessert _____
  Approximate calories _____

DAY 13: EAT ALASKAN WILD SALMON DAY

Alaskan wild salmon is among the cleanest fish with the highest levels of omega-3 fatty acids. Find a local fish market and buy these treasures. Don't get farm-raised fish—get the real thing. People who eat fish on a regular basis have a lower incidence of heart and brain problems.

- Exercise _____ (percent of targeted thirty-minute exercise accomplished)
- Supplements _____ (yes or no)
- Meditation _____ (time spent; target twelve minutes a day)
- New learning _____ (what new piece of information or new skill did you learn today?)
- What I ate today (list the food and approximate calories you ate today)
  Breakfast _____
  Snack _____
  Lunch _____
  Snack _____
  Dinner _____
  Dessert _____
  Approximate calories _____

DAY 14: GO ANT HUNTING

ANTs (automatic negative thoughts) can infest and ruin your day-to-day life. Today go hunting for these creatures with a newly acquired internal anteater. Whenever you feel sad, mad, or nervous, write out the automatic negative thought, and have your anteater talk back to them. You do not have to believe every thought you have.

- Exercise _____ (percent of targeted thirty-minute exercise accomplished)
- Supplements _____ (yes or no)
- Meditation _____ (time spent; target twelve minutes a day)
- New learning _____ (what new piece of information or new skill did you learn today?)
- What I ate today (list the food and approximate calories you ate today)
  Breakfast _____
  Snack _____
  Lunch _____
  Snack _____
  Dinner _____
  Dessert _____
  Approximate calories _____

DAY 15: COMEDY DAY

Make a concerted effort to laugh a lot today. Visit joke websites, go to see a comedy, or go to a comedy club. Laughter produces a specific set of brain chemicals that nourish hope and our immune system.

- Exercise _____ (percent of targeted thirty-minute exercise accomplished)
- Supplements _____ (yes or no)
- Meditation _____ (time spent; target twelve minutes a day)
- New learning _____ (what new piece of information or new skill did you learn today?)
- What I ate today (list the food and approximate calories you ate today)
  Breakfast _____
  Snack _____
  Lunch _____
  Snack _____
  Dinner _____
  Dessert _____
  Approximate calories _____

Over time keep up this schedule. Make caring for your brain an important part of your everyday life. Remember, one of the main goals of this book is to teach you how to love, honor, and respect your brain. It is the best part of you and can stay healthy as long as you take great care of it.

Blessings to you, your brain, and the brains of those you love!

APPENDIX

WHY SPECT

What Brain SPECT Imaging Can Tell Clinicians and Patients That They Cannot Obtain Elsewhere

If we agree that mental disorders and difficult behaviors may be related to functional problems in the brain, then a logical next step is clearly to consider *physically evaluating the brain itself* when faced with people who struggle with complex problems or are unresponsive to our best diagnostic and treatment efforts. Why are psychiatrists the only physicians who rarely look at the organ they treat?

It is time to change this situation. Amen Clinics, Inc. (ACI) has provided leadership and understanding on the clinical use of brain imaging in psychiatry. Over the past fifteen years ACI has built the world's largest database of brain scans related to emotional, learning, and behavioral problems. The study we do is called brain SPECT imaging. *SPECT* stands for "single photon emission computed tomography." It is a nuclear medicine procedure widely used to study heart, liver, thyroid, bone, and brain problems. Brain SPECT imaging is a proven, reliable measure of cerebral blood flow. Because brain activity is directly related to blood flow, SPECT effectively shows us the patterns of activity in the brain. SPECT allows physicians to look deep inside the brain to observe three things: areas of the brain that work well, areas that work too hard, and areas that do not work hard enough. ACI has performed more than thirty thousand scans on patients from age ten months to 101 years and has also scanned many normal, "healthy brain" individuals as well.

The procedure guidelines of the Society of Nuclear Medicine list the evaluation of suspected brain trauma, evaluation of patients with suspected dementia, presurgical location of seizures, and the detection and evaluation of cerebral vascular disease as common indications for brain SPECT. The guidelines also say that many additional indications appear promising. At ACI, because of our experience, we have added the indications of violence, substance abuse, the subtypes of ADD, anxiety and depression, and complex or resistant psychiatric problems for brain SPECT imaging.

An important question for today's mental health clinicians is, When and why would I order a SPECT study for my patients or get one for myself or loved one? My purpose in this appendix is to answer this question and to point out some of the benefits and caveats for using this powerful tool.

BENEFITS OF BRAIN SPECT IMAGING

A SPECT scan can provide distinct benefits to clinicians, to the patient, and to his or her family.

FIRST, THE BENEFITS FOR PHYSICIANS AND CLINICIANS:

1. A SPECT scan can show:
   a. Areas of the brain implicated in specific problems, such as the prefrontal cortex with executive function and the medial temporal lobes with long-term memory storage.
   b. Unexpected findings that may be contributing to the presenting problem(s), such as toxicity, potential areas of seizure activity, or past brain trauma.
   c. Potential seizure activity, in many cases more accurately seen by SPECT than by standard EEG, especially in the areas of the medial temporal lobe. There are more than forty-one studies with more than thirteen hundred patients on SPECT and epilepsy. See www.amenclinic.com for references.
   d. Targeted areas for treatment, such as overactive basal ganglia or anterior cingulate gyrus (seen on anxiety and OCD spectrum disorders), or underactive temporal lobe (seen in seizure disorders and trauma).

e. Specific effects of medication on the brain to help guide us in adjusting dosages or augmenting treatment. Often patients report that SSRIs are helpful but also cause decreased motivation or memory problems, seen as decreased prefrontal or temporal lobe activity on SPECT.

f. Changes in brain function with treatment, improved or worsened. You can review many before-and-after scans at www.amenclinic. com.

2. The image occurs at the time of injection and outside the imaging camera, which gives SPECT several significant advantages. Most notably, we are able to sedate people after they have been injected so that they can lie still for the scan, which is often difficult for hyperactive or autistic children or demented adults. (Motion artifact ruins the scan in all of these imaging techniques.)

3. A SPECT scan can provide explanations for refractory symptoms and help clinicians ask better and more targeted questions (such as about toxic exposure, brain injuries, anoxia, inflammation, or infections that patients may have denied or forgotten).

4. A SPECT scan can help us to avoid prescribing treatments that make the problem worse, such as unnecessarily stimulating an already overactive brain or calming an underactive one.

5. A SPECT scan can help to evaluate risk for dementia—the brain starts to change long before people show symptoms. There is usually a loss of 30 percent of hippocampal tissue before symptoms occur. Using autopsy data in fifty-four patients, F. J. Bonte reported that brain SPECT had a positive predictive value for Alzheimer's disease of 92 percent.

6. A SPECT scan can also help to differentiate among types of dementia. Early in the disease, Alzheimer's, frontal temporal lobe dementia, Lewy Body dementia, multi-infarct dementia each have their own patterns. There are over eighty-three studies with more than 4,500 patients on this subject. See www.amenclinic.com for references.

7. A SPECT scan helps clinicians understand the rationale for using certain medications (such as anticonvulsants to stabilize temporal lobe function or calm focal areas of marked hyperactivity; or stimulants to

enhance decreased prefrontal perfusion; or SSRIs to calm basal ganglia and anterior cingulate hyperactivity).

8. A SPECT scan can identify specific areas of the brain affected by trauma, better target treatment, and help deal with insurance, legal, and rehabilitation issues. There are more than thirty-eight studies on brain trauma with more than thirteen hundred patients. See www.amenclinic.com for references.

9. A SPECT scan can often identify specific factors contributing to relapse in recovering alcoholics, substance abusers, eating disordered people, or sexual addicts. For example, the patient may have suffered an injury to the prefrontal cortex or temporal lobes or have overactivity in the anterior cingulate gyrus, basal ganglia, limbic system, or prefrontal cortex, each of which could indicate a comorbid disorder that could contribute to the relapsing behavior and would require treatment.

10. A SPECT scan is also useful in determining if further adjustment of medication is needed. Scans of patients on medication will reveal areas of the brain still overactive or underactive.

BENEFITS OF SPECT BRAIN IMAGING FOR PATIENTS AND THEIR FAMILIES:

1. A SPECT scan helps develop a deeper understanding of the problem, resulting in reduced shame, guilt, stigma, and self-loathing. This understanding can promote self-forgiveness, often the first step in healing. Patients can see that their problems are, at least in part, medical and physical.

2. A SPECT scan allows patients to see a physical representation of their problems that is accurate and reliable, and that helps to increase compliance—pictures are powerful. It can influence a patient's willingness and ability to accept and adhere to the treatment program. They can better understand that not taking medication for anxiety, depression, rage, or ADD is similar to not wearing the "correct" prescription glasses.

3. A SPECT scan helps families understand that permanent brain damage from an injury will not get better, so that they can better accept the condition and provide accordingly.

4. A SPECT scan shows substance abusers the damage they have done to their own brain, thus helping to decrease denial, provide motivation for treatment, and support perseverance in sobriety.

5. A SPECT scan shows patients how treatments have impacted (improved or worsened) their brain function.

6. A SPECT scan helps motivate abusive spouses to follow medication protocols by showing them that there is a physical abnormality contributing to their problems.

7. A SPECT scan is useful for cancer patients suffering from a "chemotherapy toxic brain." It gives them insight into their cognitive struggles and also helps their doctors see the neurophysiological and emotional effects of cancer and its treatment.

8. A SPECT scan can help take modern psychopharmacology from mystery and unknown consequences to reality and more predictable outcomes.

9. A SPECT scan allows patients to understand why specific treatments are indicated, which medications are likely to be most helpful, and what other interventions may be indicated.

WHAT A SPECT SCAN CANNOT PROVIDE

Despite the many benefits that might be derived from a SPECT scan, there are clearly some things that it cannot provide. For example, a SPECT scan cannot:

1. Give a diagnosis in the absence of clinical information
2. Give the date of a head injury, infection, or toxic exposure
3. Assess or evaluate IQ
4. Assess or evaluate the guilt, innocence, motivation, or sanity of a criminal defendant
5. Guarantee a perfect diagnosis, or a cure

HOW SPECT DIFFERS FROM MRI

A SPECT scan is similar to an MRI study in that both can show three-dimensional images and "slices" of the brain. But whereas MRI shows the *physical anatomy* of the brain, SPECT shows brain *functional activity*. That is,

SPECT yields images showing where the brain is functioning well, where it is working too hard, and where it is not working hard enough. A newer version of MRI, functional MRI or "fMRI," is also capable of showing brain activity and is used extensively in scientific research on brain function. fMRI shows instantaneous neural activity so you can see, for example, how the brain responds to a specific stimulus event. With SPECT we see brain activity averaged over a few minutes so it is better at showing the brain doing everyday activities such as concentrating, meditating, reading, and the like. PET, another nuclear imaging technique, is very similar to SPECT but is slower and more costly.

ENSURING HIGH-QUALITY SPECT IMAGES

Although a SPECT scan is simple from the patient's perspective, it takes considerable skill and experience to dependably generate accurate brain SPECT images suitable for psychiatric applications. Equally important is the need for total consistency in imaging techniques among patients so that results are quantifiable, repeatable, and consistent.

Here are some of the factors that need to be considered in SPECT scans.

VARIABILITY OF TECHNIQUE ISSUES

Processing protocols need to be standardized and optimized. Motion can ruin a scan, so it is important that there be *no motion* on the scan. It's necessary to know how to identify and deal with image artifacts and other sophisticated technical issues.

VARIABILITY OF CAMERAS

Multiheaded cameras are clearly superior, as they can scan much faster. It takes an hour to do a scan on a single-headed camera, thirty minutes on a dual-headed camera, and fifteen minutes on a triple-headed camera.

EXPERIENCE OF READERS

At the Amen Clinics, we have developed a standardized reading technique for which we have documented high inter- and intra-rater reliability.

IMAGE DISPLAY

Scans must be clear, understandable, easily illustrative of brain function, and available to the patient on a timely basis. We believe our 3D rendering software makes the scans easy for professionals, patients, and families to understand.

DRUGS

Scans can be affected by a number of substances that need to be controlled for, such as medications, street drugs, and caffeine.

All of the above issues have been addressed at the Amen Clinics by carefully standardized procedures for all our SPECT scans.

COMMON CONCERNS

Concern: Because of its low resolution, a SPECT scan is commonly said to be a "poor man's PET study."

Response: With multiheaded cameras, SPECT has the same resolution as PET with considerably lower cost, better insurance coverage, greater availability, and fewer image artifacts. Also, it is an easier procedure to do. SPECT provides more than adequate resolution for our applications.

Concern: What about radiation exposure, especially in children?

Response: The average radiation exposure for one SPECT scan is 0.7 rem (similar to a nuclear bone scan or brain CAT scan) and is a safe procedure, according to the guidelines established by the American Academy of Neurology. These other procedures are routinely ordered for many common medical conditions (such as bone fractures or head trauma), further suggesting that the levels of radiation exposure are generally acceptable in medical practice. Ineffective treatment of psychiatric illness has many more risks than the low levels of radiation associated with a SPECT scan.

Concern: What is normal?

Response: In the SPECT literature over the past twenty years, more than forty-three studies have looked at "normal" issues in over 2,450 patients, including 150 children from birth on. (See www.amenclinic.com for references.) These do not include the thousands of control subjects used in studies of specific neurological and psychiatric conditions. C. Chiron, et al., reported that at birth, cortical regional cerebral blood flow (rCBF) was lower than for adults. After birth, it increased by five or six years of age to values 50 to 85 percent higher than those for adults, thereafter decreasing to reach adult levels between fifteen and nineteen years. At the age of three, however, children had the same relative blood flow patterns as adults. Other common findings in normal studies suggest that women have generally higher perfusion than men and that age, drug abuse, and smoking have a negative effect on rCBF.

Concern: Some physicians say, "I don't need a scan for diagnosis. I can tell clinically."

Response: Often well-trained physicians can tell clinically. But they order a SPECT scan when they are confused, the patient hasn't responded to their best treatment, or the patient's situation is complicated.

Concern: What about the lack of reproducibility?

Response: A paper by Javier Villanueva-Meyer, M.D., et al., elegantly answers this question, showing that there is less than 3 percent variability in SPECT scans over time for the same activity. Our own clinical experience, scanning people sequentially and sometimes twelve years apart, is that SPECT patterns are the same unless you do something to change the brain. SPECT is a reproducible and reliable method for sequential evaluation.

CONCLUSION

At the Amen Clinics we feel that our experience with more than thirty thousand brain SPECT scans over fifteen years guides us in being the best in the world for brain SPECT imaging.

COMMON QUESTIONS ABOUT BRAIN SPECT IMAGING

Here are several common questions and answers about brain SPECT imaging.

Will the SPECT study give me an accurate diagnosis? No. A SPECT study by itself will not give a diagnosis. SPECT studies help clinicians understand more about the specific function of your brain. Each person's brain is unique, which may lead to unique responses to medicine or therapy. Diagnoses about specific conditions are made through a combination of clinical history, a personal interview, information from families, diagnostic checklists, SPECT studies, and other neuropsychological tests. No study is "a doctor in a box" that can give accurate diagnoses on individual patients.

Why are SPECT studies ordered? Some of the common reasons include:

1. Evaluating memory problems and dementia and distinguishing among different types of dementia and pseudodementia (depression that looks like dementia)
2. Evaluating seizure activity
3. Evaluating blood vessel diseases, such as stroke
4. Evaluating the effects of mild, moderate, and severe head trauma
5. Suspicion of underlying organic brain condition, such as seizure activity contributing to behavioral disturbance, prenatal trauma, or exposure to toxins
6. Evaluating atypical or unresponsive aggressive behavior
7. Determining extent of brain impairment caused by the drug or alcohol abuse
8. Typing anxiety, depression, and attention deficit disorders when clinical presentation is not clear
9. Evaluating people who are atypical or resistant to treatment

Do I need to be off medication before the study? This question must be answered individually between you and your doctor. In general, it is better to be off medications until they are out of your system, but this is not always practical or advisable. If the study is done while you are on medication, let the technician know so that when the physician reads the study, he will include that information in the interpretation of the scan. In general, we recommend that patients try to be off stimulants at least four days before the first scan and remain off of them until after the second scan if one is ordered. It is generally not practical to stop medications such as Prozac because they last in the body for four to six weeks. Check with your specific doctor for recommendations.

What should I do the day of the scan? On the day of the scan decrease or eliminate your caffeine intake and try not to take cold medication or aspirin. (If you do, please write it down on the intake form.) Eat as you normally would.

Are there any side effects or risks to the study? The study does not involve a dye, and people do not have allergic reactions to it. The possibility exists, although in a very small percentage of patients, of a mild rash, facial redness and edema, fever, and a transient increase in blood pressure. The amount of radiation exposure from one brain SPECT study is approximately the same as from one abdominal X-ray.

How is the SPECT procedure done? The patient is placed in a quiet room and a small intravenous line is started. The patient remains quiet for approximately ten minutes with his or her eyes open to allow their mental state to equilibrate to the environment. The imaging agent is then injected through the IV. After another short period of time, the patient lies on a table, and the SPECT camera rotates around his or her head. (The patient does not go into a tube.) The time on the table is approximately fifteen minutes. If a concentration study is ordered, the patient returns on another day.

Are there alternatives to having a SPECT study? In our opinion, SPECT is the most clinically useful study of brain function. There are other studies, such as electroencephalograms (EEGs), positron emission tomography (PET), and functional MRIs (fMRI). PET studies and fMRI are considerably more costly and are performed mostly in the research setting. EEGs, in our opinion, do not provide enough information about the deep structures of the brain to be as helpful as SPECT studies.

Does insurance cover the cost of SPECT studies? Reimbursement by insurance companies varies according to your plan. It is often a good idea to check with the insurance company ahead of time to see if it is a covered benefit.

Is the use of brain SPECT imaging accepted in the medical community? Brain SPECT studies are widely recognized as an effective tool for evaluating brain function in seizures, strokes, dementia, and head trauma. There are literally hundreds of research articles on these topics. In our clinic, based on our experience for over a decade, we have developed this technology further to evaluate aggression and nonresponsive psychiatric conditions. Unfortunately, many physicians do not fully understand the application of SPECT imaging and may tell you that the technology is experimental, but more than one thousand physicians and mental health professionals in the United States have referred patients to us for scans.

GLOSSARY

Acetylcholine (ACh)   a neurotransmitter involved in memory formation, mostly excitatory; it has been implicated in problems with muscles, Alzheimer's disease, and learning

Acetyl-L-carnitine (ALC)   an amino acid involved in the transport of fatty acids into the cells' mitochondria for the purpose of producing energy; may be helpful in preventing strokes and heart attacks

Alpha-lipoic acid (ALA)   a powerful antioxidant that increases the potency of many other antioxidants

Alzheimer's disease (AD)   the most common form of dementia; results from beta-amyloid production and neurofibrillary tangles

Antioxidant   a substance that helps prevent damage from free radical formation

Apolipoprotein E (apoE) gene   a gene involved in the development, maturation, and repair of cell membranes of neurons; helps regulate the amount of cholesterol and triglycerides in nerve cell membranes. There are three versions of the apoE gene: E2, E3, and E4. It is the last one that is the culprit—the apoE4 gene increases the risk of Alzheimer's disease, as well as a number of other illnesses.

Axon   usually, a long process that projects from a cell body to connect with other cells

Central nervous system (CNS)   a body system composed of the spinal cord and parts of the brain, brainstem, thalamus, basal ganglia, cerebellum, and cerebral cortex

Coenzyme Q10 (CoQ10)   an enzyme that lives inside the mitochondria, and helps convert oxygen into usable cellular energy called ATP

Dendrite a structure that branches out from a cell body and serves as the main receiver of signals from other nerve cells; it functions as the "antenna" of the neuron

Dopamine a neurotransmitter involved in attention, motor movements, and motivation; has been implicated in Parkinson's disease, attention deficit disorder, addictions, depression, and schizophrenia

fMRI a brain scan that uses powerful magnets to look at brain blood flow and activity patterns

Free radical a highly toxic substance, produced when oxygen combines with other molecules, that must be neutralized by antioxidants or it will cause damage to cells

Gamma-aminobutyric acid (GABA) an inhibitory neurotransmitter involved in calming brain function; has been implicated in seizures, bipolar disorder, anxiety, and pain

Ginkgo biloba an herb from the Chinese ginkgo tree that is known to improve circulation and blood flow; has been shown to be helpful in dementia

Glutamate an excitatory (stimulating) neurotransmitter

Hippocampus the part of the inside of the temporal lobes that facilitates memory function

Homocysteine an amino acid that when elevated increases the risk of Alzheimer's disease, stroke, and heart disease

Long-term potentiation (LTP) the process of invigorating (or potentiating) neurons to do their job over a long period of time; accomplished through the repetition of an act, which causes actual physical changes in neurons and their synapses

Magnetic resonance imaging (MRI) a brain scan that uses powerful magnets to look at the physical structure of organs

Melatonin a naturally produced hormone that helps regulate sleep-wake cycles

Memantine (Axura) an NMDA antagonist; a drug that may have protective effects on certain glutamate receptors against the overproduction of glutamate, which is toxic in large amounts

Myelin the whitish protein covering of a neuron

Myelination the act of laying down myelin onto neurons

Nerve growth factor (NGF) a growth factor in the brain that promotes the regeneration of nerve cells after injury

Neurogenesis the growth of new neurons

Neurotransmitter a chemical that is released from one neuron at the presynaptic nerve terminal (the end of an axon), then crosses the synapse, where it may be accepted by the next neuron (on the dendrites) at specialized sites called receptors; there are many different neurotransmitters, such as acetylcholine, serotonin, dopamine, and norepinephrine

Neuron a nerve cell

Nonsteroidal anti-inflammatory drug (NSAID) a common pain-killing medication that works in part by decreasing inflammation and thinning the blood; some NSAIDs also appear to block the production of beta-amyloid

Norepinephrine a neurotransmitter involved in mood, concentration, and motivation; thought to be associated with problems of attention, depression, and anxiety

Parkinson's disease (PD) a disease caused by loss of neurons that produce the neurotransmitter dopamine in a part of the brainstem called the substantia nigra; often associated with a tremor, slowed movements, and rigidity; often associated with dementia after three years

Positron emission tomography (PET) a brain scan that uses isotopes to look at glucose metabolism and activity patterns in the brain

Serotonin (5-HT) a neurotransmitter involved in mood, flexibility, and shifting attention; often involved in depression, obsessive-compulsive disorder, eating disorders, sleep disturbances, and pain

Single photon emission computed tomography (SPECT) a brain scan that uses isotopes to look at blood flow and activity patterns in the brain

Statin a drug to lower cholesterol

Synapse a junction formed between nerve cells where the presynaptic terminal of an axon comes into "contact" with the dendrite's postsynaptic membrane of another neuron; there are two types of synapses, electrical and chemical

Synaptic plasticity the ability of a synapse to change in order to more efficiently signal other neurons

Vinpocetine a substance derived from an extract of the common periwinkle plant (*Vinca minor*); a cerebral vasodilator, increasing blood flow to the brain; may be helpful for Alzheimer's disease, vascular dementia, and cardiovascular illnesses

REFERENCES AND FURTHER READING

CHAPTER 1

Johnson, D. L., et al., "Cerebral Blood Flow and Personality: A Positron Emission Tomography Study." *American Journal of Psychiatry* 156, no. 2 (February 1999): 252–57.

Keightley, M. L., et al., "Personality Influences Limbic-Cortical Interactions During Sad Mood Induction," *Neuroimage* 20, no. 4 (December 2003): 2031–39.

Kumari, V., et al., "Personality Predicts Brain Responses to Cognitive Demands," *Journal of Neuroscience* 24, no. 47 (November 24, 2004): 10636–41.

Sugiura, M., et al., "Correlation Between Human Personality and Neural Activity in Cerebral Cortex," *Neuroimage* 11, no. 5, pt. 1 (May 2000): 541–46.

Turner, R. M., et al., "Brain Function and Personality in Normal Males: A SPECT Study Using Statistical Parametric Mapping," *Neuroimage* 19, no. 3 (July 2003): 1145–62.

Youn, T., et al., "Relationship Between Personality Trait and Regional Cerebral Glucose Metabolism Assessed with Positron Emission Tomography," *Biological Psychology* 60, no. 2–3 (September 2002): 109–20.

CHAPTER 2

Alptekin, K., et al., "Tc-99m HMPAO Brain Perfusion SPECT in Drug-Free Obsessive-Compulsive Patients Without Depression," *Psychiatry Research* 107, no. 1 (July 1, 2001): 51–56.

Catafau, A. M., et al., "Regional Cerebral Blood Flow Pattern in Normal Young and

Aged Volunteers: A 99mTc-HMPAO SPET study," *European Journal of Nuclear Medicine* 23, no. 10 (October 1996): 1329–37.

Chiron, C., et al., "Changes in Regional Cerebral Blood Flow During Brain Maturation in Children and Adolescents," *Journal of Nuclear Medicine* 33, no. 5 (May 1992): 696–703.

George, M. S., et al., "Elevated Frontal Cerebral Blood Flow in Gilles de la Tourette Syndrome: A 99Tcm-HMPAO SPECT Study," *Psychiatry Research* 45, no. 3 (November 1992): 143–51.

Goto, R., et al., "A Comparison of Tc-99m HMPAO Brain SPECT Images of Young and Aged Normal Individuals," *Annals of Nuclear Medicine* 12, no. 6 (December 1998): 333–39.

Lacerda, A. L., et al., "Elevated Thalamic and Prefrontal Regional Cerebral Blood Flow in Obsessive-Compulsive Disorder: A SPECT Study," *Psychiatry Research* 123, no. 2 (June 30, 2003): 125–34.

Machlin, S. R., et al., "Elevated Medial-Frontal Cerebral Blood Flow in Obsessive-Compulsive Patients: A SPECT Study," *American Journal of Psychiatry* 148, no. 9 (September 1991): 1240–42.

Mena, Francisco J., et al., "Children Normal HMPAO Brain SPECT," *Alasbimn Journal* 1, no. 1 (September 1998); http://www.alasbimnjournal.cl/revistas/1/children.htm.

Saxena, S., R. G. Bota, and A. L. Brody, "Brain-Behavior Relationships in Obsessive-Compulsive Disorder," *Seminars in Clinical Neuropsychiatry* 6, no. 2 (April 2001): 82–101.

CHAPTER 3

Neuroscience for Kids
  http://faculty.washington.edu/chudler/neurok.html
The Franklin Institute Online
  http://sln.fi.edu/qa97/spotlight5/spotlight5.html

CHAPTER 4

Abdel-Dayem, H. M., et al., "SPECT Brain Perfusion Abnormalities in Mild or Moderate Traumatic Brain Injury," *Clinical Nuclear Medicine* 23, no. 5 (May 1998): 309–17.

Abu-Judeh, H. H., et al., "SPECT Brain Perfusion Imaging in Mild Traumatic Brain Injury Without Loss of Consciousness and Normal Computed Tomography," *Nuclear Medicine Communications* 20, no. 6 (June 1999): 305–10.

Barnes, B. C., et al., "Concussion History in Elite Male and Female Soccer Players," *American Journal of Sports Medicine* 26, no. 3 (May–June 1998): 433–38.

Bergsneider, M., et al., "Metabolic Recovery Following Human Traumatic Brain Injury Based on FDG-PET: Time Course and Relationship to Neurological Disability," *Journal of Head Trauma Rehabilitation* 16, no. 2 (April 2001): 135–48.

Babbs, C. F., "Biomechanics of Heading a Soccer Ball: Implications for Player Safety," *Scientific World Journal* 1 (August 8, 2001): 281–322.

Boll, T. J., and J. Barth, "Mild Head Injury," *Psychiatric Development* 1, no. 3 (Autumn 1983): 263–75.

Furtak, J., K. Chmielowski, and J. K. Podgorski, "Epidemiology, Diagnosis and Prognosis in the Clinical Syndrome of Brain Concussion," *Neurologia i neurochirurgia polska* 30, no. 4 (July–August 1996): 625–30.

Goshen, E., et al., "The Role of 99Tcm-HMPAO Brain SPECT in Paediatric Traumatic Brain Injury," *Nuclear Medicine Communications* 17, no. 5 (May 1996): 418–22.

Jacobs, A., et al., "One-Year Follow-up of Technetium-99m-HMPAO SPECT in Mild Head Injury," *Journal of Nuclear Medicine* 37, no. 10 (October 1996): 1605–09.

Kemp, P. M., et al., "Cerebral Perfusion and Psychometric Testing in Military Amateur Boxers and Controls," *Journal of Neurology, Neurosurgery and Psychiatry* 59, no. 4 (October 1995): 368–74.

Kirkendall, D. T., S. E. Jordan, and W. E. Garrett, "Heading and Head Injuries in Soccer," *Sports Medicine* 31, no. 5 (2001): 369–86.

Lovell, M. R., et al., "Recovery from Mild Concussion in High School Athletes," *Journal of Neurosurgery* 98, no. 2 (February 2003): 296–301.

Massagli, T. L., et al., "Psychiatric Illness After Mild Traumatic Brain Injury in Children," *Archive of Physical Medicine and Rehabilitation* 85, no. 9 (September 2004): 1428–34.

Matser, E. J., et al., "Neuropsychological Impairment in Amateur Soccer Players," *Journal of the American Medical Association* 282, no. 10 (September 8, 1999): 971–73.

Tysvaer, A. T., O. V. Storli, N. I. Bachen, "Soccer Injuries to the Brain. A Neurologic and Electroencephalographic Study of Former Players," *Acta Neurologica Scandinavica* 80, no. 2 (August 1989): 151–56.

CHAPTER 5

Amen, D. G., *Change Your Brain, Change Your Life* (New York: Three Rivers Press, 2000).

Bogg, T., and B. W. Roberts, "Conscientiousness and Health-Related Behaviors: A Meta-Analysis of the Leading Behavioral Contributors to Mortality," *Psychological Bulletin* 130, no. 6 (November 2004): 887–919.

Kolb, B., and I. Wishaw, *Fundamentals of Human Neuropsychology* (New York: W.H. Freeman and Co., 2003).

Miller, B., and J. Cummings, *The Human Frontal Lobes* (New York: Guilford Press, 1998).

CHAPTER 6

Amen, D. G., *Healing ADD* (New York: Putnam, 2001).

Amen, D. G., and L. C. Routh, *Healing Anxiety and Depression* (New York: Putnam, 2003).

Diagnostic and Statistical Manual of Mental Disorders IV-TR (New York: American Psychiatric Association, 2000).

CHAPTER 7

Amen, D. G., J. C. Wu, and B. L. Carmichael, "The Clinical Use of Brain SPECT Imaging in Neuropsychiatry," *Alasbimn Journal* 5, no. 19 (January 2003); http://www2.alasbimnjournal.cl/alasbimn/CDA/sec_b/0,1206,SCID%253D3 212,00.html.

Amen, D. G., "Why Don't Psychiatrists Look at the Brain: The Case for the Greater Use of SPECT Imaging in Neuropsychiatry," *Neuropsychiatry Reviews* 2, no. 1 (February 2001): 19–21.

———, "Brain SPECT Imaging in Psychiatry," *Primary Psychiatry* 5, no. 8 (August 1998): 83–90.

———, "Brain SPECT Imaging and ADD," in *Understanding, Diagnosing, and Treating AD/HD in Children and Adolescents: An Integrative Approach,* edited by J. A. Incorvaia, et al. (Northvale, N.J.: Jason Aronson, 1999): 183–96.

———, "New Directions in the Theory, Diagnosis, and Treatment of Mental Disorders: The Use of SPECT Imaging in Everyday Clinical Practice," in *The Neuropsychology of Mental Disorders,* edited by L.F. Koziol and C.E. Stout (Springfield, Ill.: Charles C. Thomas, 1994): 286–311.

Wu, J. C., D. G. Amen, and S. Bracha, "Functional Neuroimaging in Clinical Practice," in *The Comprehensive Textbook of Psychiatry,* edited by H.I. Kaplan and B.J. Sadock (Philadelphia: Lippincott Williams and Wilkins, 2000).

CHAPTER 8

Amen, D. G., *Change Your Brain, Change Your Life* (New York: Three Rivers Press, 2000).

———, *Healing the Hardware of the Soul* (New York: Free Press, 2002).

————, "Three Years on Clomipramine: Before and After Brain SPECT Study," *Annals of Clinical Psychiatry* 9, no. 2 (1997): 113–16.

Carey, P. D., et al., "Single Photon Emission Computed Tomography (SPECT) of Anxiety Disorders Before and After Treatment with Citalopram," *BMC Psychiatry* 4, no. 1 (October 2004): 30.

Catafau, A. M., et al., "SPECT Mapping of Cerebral Activity Changes Induced by Repetitive Transcranial Magnetic Stimulation in Depressed Patients. A Pilot Study," *Psychiatry Research* 106, no. 3 (May 30, 2001): 151–60.

Dormehl, I. C., et al., "SPECT Monitoring of Improved Cerebral Blood Flow During Long-term Treatment of Elderly Patients with Nootropic Drugs," *Clinical Nuclear Medicine* 24, no. 1 (January 1999): 29–34.

Furmark, T., et al., "Common Changes in Cerebral Blood Flow in Patients with Social Phobia Treated with Citalopram or Cognitive-Behavioral Therapy," *Archives of General Psychiatry* 59, no. 5 (May 2002): 425–33.

Golden, Z. L., et al., "Improvement in Cerebral Metabolism in Chronic Brain Injury After Hyperbaric Oxygen Therapy," *International Journal of Neuroscience* 112, no. 2 (February 2002): 119–31.

Holthoff, V. A., et al., "Changes in Regional Cerebral Perfusion in Depression. SPECT Monitoring of Response to Treatment," *Nervenarzt* 70, no. 7 (July 1999): 620–26.

Laatsch, L., et al., "Impact of Cognitive Rehabilitation Therapy on Neuropsychological Impairments as Measured by Brain Perfusion SPECT: A Longitudinal Study," *Brain Injury* 11, no. 12 (December 1997): 851–63.

Lansing, K., D. G. Amen, and C. Hanks, "High Resolution Brain SPECT Imaging and EMDR in Police Officers with PTSD," *Journal of Neuropsychiatry* (2005).

Levin, P., S. Lazrove, and B. van der Kolk, "What Psychological Testing and Neuroimaging Tell Us About the Treatment of Posttraumatic Stress Disorder by Eye Movement Desensitization and Reprocessing," *Journal of Anxiety Disorders* 13, no. 1–2 (January–April 1999): 159–72.

Martin, S. D., et al., "Brain Blood Flow Changes in Depressed Patients Treated with Interpersonal Psychotherapy or Venlafaxine Hydrochloride: Preliminary Findings," *Archives of General Psychiatry* 58, no. 7 (July 2001): 641–48.

Paquette, V., et al., " 'Change the Mind and You Change the Brain': Effects of Cognitive-Behavioral Therapy on the Neural Correlates of Spider Phobia," *Neuroimage* 18, no. 2 (February 2003): 401–09.

Santos, R. F., et al., "Cognitive Performance, SPECT, and Blood Viscosity in Elderly Non-demented People Using Ginkgo Biloba," *Pharmacopsychiatry* 36, no. 4 (July 2003): 127–33.

Shi, X. Y., "Cerebral Perfusion SPECT Imaging for Assessment of the Effect of

Hyperbaric Oxygen Therapy on Patients with Postbrain Injury Neural Status," *Chinese Journal of Traumatology* 6, no. 6 (December 2003): 346–49.

Vasile, R. G., et al., "Changes in Regional Cerebral Blood Flow Following Light Treatment for Seasonal Affective Disorder: Responders Versus Nonresponders," *Biological Psychiatry* 42, no. 11 (December 1, 1997): 1000–05.

CHAPTER 9

Mental Health: A Report of the Surgeon General, http://www.surgeongeneral.gov/library/mentalhealth/home.html

Ortberg, J., *Everybody's Normal Till You Get to Know Them* (Grand Rapids, Mich.: Zondervan, 2003).

CHAPTER 10

Chang, L., et al., "Effect of Ecstasy [3,4-methylenedioxymethamphetamine (MDMA)] on Cerebral Blood Flow: A Co-registered SPECT and MRI Study," *Psychiatry Research* 98, no. 1 (February 28, 2000): 15–28.

De Mendelssohn, A., S. Kasper, and J. Tauscher, "Neuroimaging in Substance Abuse Disorders," *Nervenarzt* 75, no. 7 (July 2004): 651–62.

Demir, B., et al., "Regional Cerebral Blood Flow and Neuropsychological Functioning in Early and Late Onset Alcoholism," *Psychiatry Research* (June 2002): 115–25.

Dupont, R. M., et al., "Single Photon Emission Computed Tomography with Iodoamphetamine-123 and Neuropsychological Studies in Long-term Abstinent Alcoholics," *Psychiatry Research* 67, no. 2 (July 1996): 99–111.

Erbas, B., et al., "Regional Cerebral Blood Flow Changes in Chronic Alcoholism Using Tc-99m HMPAO SPECT. Comparison with CT Parameters," *Clinical Nuclear Medicine* 17, no. 2 (February 1992): 123–27.

Ernst, T., et al., "Cerebral Perfusion Abnormalities in Abstinent Cocaine Abusers: A Perfusion MRI and SPECT Study," *Psychiatry Research* 99, no. 2 (August 28, 2000): 63–74.

Gerra, G., et al., "Regional Cerebral Blood Flow and Comorbid Diagnosis in Abstinent Opioid Addicts," *Psychiatry Research* 83, no. 2 (August 26, 1998): 117–26.

Harris, G. J., et al., "Hypoperfusion of the Cerebellum and Aging Effects on Cerebral Cortex Blood Flow in Abstinent Alcoholics: A SPECT Study," *Alcoholism—Clinical and Experimental Research* 23, no. 7 (July 1999): 1219–27.

Holman, B. L., et al., "Brain Perfusion is Abnormal in Cocaine-Dependent Polydrug Users: A Study Using Technetium-99m-HMPAO and SPECT," *Journal of Nuclear Medicine* 32, no. 6 (June 1991): 1206–10.

Iyo, M., et al., "Abnormal Cerebral Perfusion in Chronic Methamphetamine

Abusers: A Study Using 99MTc-HMPAO and SPECT," *Progress in Neuropsychopharmacol and Biological Psychiatry* 21, no. 5 (July 1997): 789–96.

Kao, C. H., S. J. Wang, and S. H. Yeh, "Presentation of Regional Cerebral Blood Flow in Amphetamine Abusers by 99Tcm-HMPAO Brain SPECT," *Nuclear Medicine Communications* 15, no. 2 (February 1994): 94–98.

Kucuk, N. O., et al., "Brain SPECT Findings in Long-term Inhalant Abuse," *Nuclear Medicine Communications* 21, no. 8 (August 2000): 769–73.

Lotfi, J., and J. S. Meyer, "Cerebral Hemodynamic and Metabolic Effects of Chronic Alcoholism," *Cerebrovascular and Brain Metabolism Review* 1, no. 1 (Spring 1989): 2–25.

Mathew, R. J., et al., "Marijuana Intoxication and Brain Activation in Marijuana Smokers," *Life Sciences* 60, no. 23 (1997): 2075–89.

Miller, B. L., et al., "Neuropsychiatric Effects of Cocaine: SPECT Measurements," *Journal of Addictive Diseases* 11, no. 4 (1992): 47–58.

Okada, S., et al., "Regional Cerebral Blood Flow Abnormalities in Chronic Solvent Abusers," *Psychiatry and Clinical Neurosciences* 53, no. 3 (June 1999): 351–56.

Volkow, N. D., et al., "Decreased Brain Metabolism in Neurologically Intact Healthy Alcoholics," *American Journal of Psychiatry* 149, no. 8 (August 1992): 1016–22.

Brain Injury

Baker, B., "Head Injury Confers Alzheimer's Risk Regardless of Apo E-4 Status," *Clinical Psychiatry News* 28, no. 1 (2000).

De Deyn, P. P., et al., "From Neuronal and Vascular Impairment to Dementia," *Pharmacopsychiatry* 32 (Supp.) (1999): 17–24.

Graham, D. I., et al., "Apolipoprotein E and the Response of the Brain to Injury," *Acta Neurochirurgica* 73 (Suppl.) (1999): 89–92.

Johnstone, B., M. K. Childers, and J. Hoerner, "The Effects of Normal Ageing on Neuropsychological Functioning Following Traumatic Brain Injury," *Brain Injury* 12, no. 7 (1998): 569–76.

Jordan, B. D., et al., "Apolipoprotein E4 Associated with Chronic Traumatic Brain Injury in Boxing," *Journal of the American Medical Association* 278, no. 2 (1997): 136–40.

Kerr, M. E., and M. Kraus, "Genetics and the Central Nervous System: Apolipoprotein E and Brain Injury," *AACN Clinical Issues* 9, no. 4 (1998): 524–30.

Mayeux, R., et al., "Synergistic Effects of Traumatic Head Injury and Apolipoprotein E-4 in Patients with Alzheimer's Disease," *Neurology* 48 (1995): 555–57.

Nemetz, P. N., et al., "Traumatic Brain Injury and Time to Onset of Alzheimer's Disease: A Population-Based Study," *American Journal of Epidemiology* 149, no. 1 (1999): 32–40.

Rasmusson, D. X., et al., "Head Injury as a Risk Factor in Alzheimer's Disease," *Brain Injury* 9, no. 3 (1995): 213–19.

Salib, E., and V. Hillier, "Head Injury and the Risk of Alzheimer's Disease: A Case Control Study," *International Journal of Geriatric Psychiatry* 12 (1999): 363–68.

Shankle, W. R., and D. G. Amen, *Preventing Alzheimer's* (New York: Putnam, 2004).

Yamada, M., et al., "Prevalence and Risks of Dementia in the Japanese Population: RERF's Adult Health Study Hiroshima Subjects," *Journal of the American Geriatrics Society* 47 (1999): 189–95.

Caffeine

Field, A. S., et al., "Dietary Caffeine Consumption and Withdrawal: Confounding Variables in Quantitative Cerebral Perfusion Studies?" *Radiology* 227, no. 1 (2003): 129–35.

Hoecker, C., et al., "Caffeine Impairs Cerebral and Intestinal Blood Flow Velocity in Preterm Infants," *Pediatrics* 109, no. 5 (May 2002): 784–87.

Laurienti, P. J., et al., "Dietary Caffeine Consumption Modulates fMRI Measures," *Neuroimage* 17, no. 2 (October 2002): 751–57.

Lunt, M. J., et al., "Comparison of Caffeine-Induced Changes in Cerebral Blood Flow and Middle Cerebral Artery Blood Velocity Shows That Caffeine Reduces Middle Cerebral Artery Diameter," *Physiological Measurement* 25, no. 2 (April 2004): 467–74.

Mathew, R. J., and W. H. Wilson, "Caffeine-Induced Changes in Cerebral Circulation," *Stroke* 16, no. 5 (September–October 1985): 814–17.

Mathew, R. J., D. L. Barr, and M. L. Weinman, "Caffeine and Cerebral Blood Flow," *British Journal of Psychiatry* 143 (December 1983): 604–08.

Ragab, S., et al., "Caffeine Reduces Cerebral Blood Flow in Patients Recovering from an Ischaemic Stroke," *Age and Ageing* 33, no. 3 (May 2004): 299–303.

Nicotine

Domino, E. F., et al., "Nicotine Effects on Regional Cerebral Blood Flow in Awake, Resting Tobacco Smokers," *Synapse* 38, no. 3 (Dec. 1, 2000): 313–21.

Ghatan, P. H., et al., "Cerebral Effects of Nicotine During Cognition in Smokers and Non-smokers," *Psychopharmacology* 136, no. 2 (March 1998): 179–89.

Kubota, K., et al., "Effects of Smoking on Regional Cerebral Blood Flow in Neurologically Normal Subjects," *Stroke* 14, no. 5 (September–October 1983): 720–24.

Pergadia, M., et al., "Double-Blind Trial of the Effects of Tryptophan Depletion on Depression and Cerebral Blood Flow in Smokers," *Addictive Behaviors* 29, no. 4 (June 2004): 668–71.

Rose, J. E., et al., "PET Studies of the Influences of Nicotine on Neural Systems in Cigarette Smokers," *American Journal of Psychiatry* 160, no. 2 (February 2003): 323–33.

Yamashita, K., et al., "Effect of Smoking on Regional Cerebral Blood Flow in the Normal Aged Volunteers," *Gerontology* 34, no. 4 (1988): 199–204.

Sleep

Bliwise, D. L., "Sleep Apnea, APOE4 and Alzheimer's Disease 20 Years and Counting?" *Journal of Psychosomatic Research* 53, no. 1 (July 2002): 539–46.

Drummond, S. P., et al., "Sleep Deprivation-Induced Reduction in Cortical Functional Response to Serial Subtraction," *Neuroreport* 10, no. 18 (December 16, 1999): 3745–48.

Miller, G., "Society for Neuroscience Meeting. Brain Cells May Pay the Price for a Bad Night's Sleep," *Science* 306, no. 5699 (Nov. 12, 2004): 1126.

Spiegel, K., "Leptin Levels Are Dependent on Sleep Duration: Relationships with Sympathovagal Balance, Carbohydrate Regulation, Cortisol, and Thyrotropin," *Journal of Clinical Endocrinology and Metabolism* 89, no. 11 (November 2004): 5762–71.

Spiegel, K., et al., "Brief Communication: Sleep Curtailment in Healthy Young Men Is Associated with Decreased Leptin Levels, Elevated Ghrelin Levels, and Increased Hunger and Appetite," *Annals of Internal Medicine* 141, no. 11 (December 7, 2004): 846–50.

Tanaka, H., and S. Shirakawa, "Sleep Health, Lifestyle and Mental Health in the Japanese Elderly: Ensuring Sleep to Promote a Healthy Brain and Mind," *Journal of Psychosomatic Research* 56, no. 5 (May 2004): 465–77.

Stress

Duval, F., et al., "Increased Adrenocorticotropin Suppression Following Dexamethasone Administration in Sexually Abused Adolescents with Post-traumatic Stress Disorder," *Psychoneuroendocrinology* 29, no. 10 (November 2004): 1281–89.

Lansing, K., et al., "High Resolution Brain SPECT Imaging and EMDR with Police Officers Involved in Shootings," *Journal of Neuropsychiatry and Clinical Neuroscience* (in press).

Levin, P., S. Lazrove, and B. van der Kolk, "What Psychological Testing and Neuroimaging Tell Us About the Treatment of Posttraumatic Stress Disorder by Eye Movement Desensitization and Reprocessing," *Journal of Anxiety Disorders* 13, no. 1–2 (January–April 1999): 159–72.

Sala, M., et al., "Stress and Hippocampal Abnormalities in Psychiatric Disorders," *European Neuropsychopharmacology* 14, no. 5 (October 2004): 393–405.

Stein, M. B., et al., "Enhanced Dexamethasone Suppression of Plasma Cortisol in Adult Women Traumatized by Childhood Sexual Abuse," *Biological Psychiatry* 42, no. 8 (October 15, 1997): 680–86.

Yehuda, R., et al., "Enhanced Suppression of Cortisol Following Dexamethasone Administration in Post-traumatic Stress Disorder," *American Journal of Psychiatry* 150, no. 1 (January 1993): 83–86.

Yehuda, R., "Biology of Post-traumatic Stress Disorder," *Journal of Clinical Psychiatry* 62, supp. 17 (2001): 41–46.

CHAPTER 11

Barberger-Gateau, P., "Fish, Meat, and Risk of Dementia: Cohort Study," *British Medical Journal* 325, no. 7370 (October 26, 2002): 932–33.

Conquer, J. A., et al., "Fatty Acid Analysis of Blood Plasma of Patients with Alzheimer's Disease, Other Types of Dementia, and Cognitive Impairment," *Lipids* 35, no. 12 (December 2000): 1305–12.

Ingram, D. K., et al., "Development of Calorie Restriction Mimetics as a Pro-longevity Strategy," *Annals of the New York Academy of Science* 1019 (June 2004): 412–23.

Kim, Y. K., and A. M. Myint, "Clinical Application of Low Serum Cholesterol as an Indicator for Suicide Risk in Major Depression," *Journal of Affective Disorders* 81, no. 2 (August 2004): 161–66.

Kim, Y. K., et al., "Low Serum Cholesterol Is Correlated to Suicidality in a Korean Sample," *Acta Psychiatrica Scandinavica* 105, no. 2 (February 2002): 141–48.

Larrieu, S., et al., "Nutritional Factors and Risk of Incident Dementia in the PAQUID Longitudinal Cohort," *Journal of Nutrition, Health, and Aging* 8, no. 3 (2004): 150–54.

Liu, J., et al., "Malnutrition at Age 3 Years and Externalizing Behavior Problems at Ages 8, 11, and 17 Years," *American Journal of Psychiatry* 161, no. 11 (Nov. 2004): 2005–13.

Mattson, M. P., W. Duan, and Z. Guo, "Meal Size and Frequency Affect Neuronal Plasticity and Vulnerability to Disease: Cellular and Molecular Mechanisms," *Journal of Neurochemistry* 84, no. 3 (February 2003): 417–31.

McIlwain, H., and H. S. Bachelard, *Biochemistry and the Central Nervous System* (Edinburgh: Churchill Livingstone, 1985).

Molteni, R., et al., "A High-Fat, Refined Sugar Diet Reduces Hippocampal Brain-Derived Neurotrophic Factor, Neuronal Plasticity, and Learning," *Neuroscience* 112, no. 4 (2002): 803–14.

Roth, G. S., D. K. Ingram, and M. A. Lane, "Caloric Restriction in Primates and Relevance to Humans," *Annals of the New York Academy of Sciences* 928 (April 2001): 305–15.

Wu, A., et al., "A Saturated-Fat Diet Aggravates the Outcome of Traumatic Brain Injury on Hippocampal Plasticity and Cognitive Function by Reducing Brain-Derived Neurotrophic Factor," *Neuroscience* 119, no. 2 (2003): 368–75.

CHAPTER 12

Christakis, D. A., et al., "Early Television Exposure and Subsequent Attentional Problems in Children," *Pediatrics* 113 (April 2004): 708–13.

Diamond, M., S. Cusack, and W. Thompson, *Mental Fitness for Life: A 7 Step Guide to Healthy Aging* (Toronto: Key Porter Books, 2003).

Hancox, R. J., B. J. Milne, and R. Poulton, "Association Between Child and Adolescent Television Viewing and Adult Health: A Longitudinal Birth Cohort Study," *Lancet* 364, no. 9430 (July 17, 2004): 257–62.

Koepp, M. J., et al., "Evidence for Striatal Dopamine Release During a Video Game," *Nature* 393, no. 6682 (May 21, 1998): 266–68.

Mohammed, A. H., et al., "Environmental Enrichment and the Brain," *Progress in Brain Research* 138 (2002): 109–33.

Snowdon, D. A., "Aging and Alzheimer's Disease: Lessons from the Nun Study," *Gerontologist* 37, no. 2 (1997): 150–56.

Van Praag, H., G. Kempermann, and F. H. Gage, "Neural Consequences of Environmental Enrichment," *Native Reviews—Neuroscience* 1, no. 3 (December 2000): 191–98.

CHAPTER 13

Beatty, J. A., et al., "Physical Exercise Decreases Neuronal Activity in the Posterior Hypothalamic Area of Spontaneously Hypertensive Rats," *Journal of Applied Physiology* 11, no. 2 (October 8, 2004): 75–84.

Colcombe, S. J., et al., "Neurocognitive Aging and Cardiovascular Fitness: Recent Findings and Future Directions," *Journal of Molecular Neuroscience* 24, no. 1 (2004): 9–14.

Friedland, R. P., et al., "Patients with Alzheimer's Disease Have Reduced Activities in Midlife Compared with Healthy Control-Group Members," *Proceedings of the National Academy of Sciences* 98, no. 6 (March 13, 2001): 3440–45.

Guszkowska, M., "The Effects of Exercise on Anxiety, Depression and Mood States," *Psychiatria Polska* 38, no. 4 (July–August 2004): 611–20.

Korf, E. S., et al., "Midlife Blood Pressure and the Risk of Hippocampal Atrophy: The Honolulu Asia Aging Study," *Hypertension* 44, no. 1 (July 2004): 29–34.

Lindsay, J., et al., "Risk Factors for Alzheimer's Disease: A Prospective Analysis from the Canadian Study of Health and Aging," *American Journal of Epidemiology* 156, no. 5 (September 1, 2002): 445–53.

Lytle, M. E., et al., "Exercise Level and Cognitive Decline: The MoVIES Project," *Alzheimer Disease and Associated Disorders* 18, no. 2 (April–June 2004): 57–64.

Mattson, M. P., "Neuroprotective Signaling and the Aging Brain: Take Away My

Food and Let Me Run," *Brain Research* 886, no. 1–2 (December 15, 2000): 47–53.

Mattson, M. P., S. Maudsley, and B. Martin, "BDNF and 5-HT: A Dynamic Duo in Age-Related Neuronal Plasticity and Neurodegenerative Disorders," *Trends in Neuroscience* 27, no. 10 (October 2004): 589–94.

Molteni, R., "Exercise Reverses the Harmful Effects of Consumption of a High-Fat Diet on Synaptic and Behavioral Plasticity Associated to the Action of Brain-Derived Neurotrophic Factor," *Neuroscience* 123, no. 2 (2004): 429–40.

Vaynman, S., Z. Ying, and F. Gomez-Pinilla, "Interplay Between Brain-Derived Neurotrophic Factor and Signal Transduction Modulators in the Regulation of the Effects of Exercise on Synaptic-Plasticity," *Neuroscience* 122, no. 3 (2003): 647–57.

CHAPTER 14

Draganski, B., et al., "Neuroplasticity: Changes in Grey Matter Induced by Training," *Nature* 427, no. 6972 (January 22, 2004): 311–12.

Kolb, B., and I. Q. Whishaw, "Brain Plasticity and Behavior," *Annual Review of Psychology* 49 (1998): 43–64.

Morris, G. S., J. M. Sifft, and G. K. Khalsa, "Effect of Educational Kinesiology on Static Balance of Learning Disabled Students," *Perceptual and Motor Skills* 67, no. 1 (August 1998): 51–54.

Schlaug, G., "The Brain of Musicians. A Model for Functional and Structural Adaptation," *Annals of the New York Academy of Sciences* 930 (June 2001): 281–99.

Shaffer, R. J., "Effect of Interactive Metronome Training on Children with ADHD," *American Journal of Occupational Therapy* 55, no. 2 (March–April 2001): 155–62.

Sifft, J. M., and G. C. Khalsa, "Effect of Educational Kinesiology upon Simple Response Times and Choice Response Times," *Perceptual and Motor Skills* 73, no. 3, pt. 1 (December 1991): 1011–15.

Ungerleider, L. G., J. Doyon, and A. Karni, "Imaging Brain Plasticity During Motor Skill Learning," *Neurobiology of Learning and Memory* 78, no. 3 (November 2002): 553–64.

CHAPTER 15

Abramov, L. A., "Sexual Life and Sexual Frigidity Among Women Developing Acute Myocardial Infarction," *Psychosomatic Medicine* 38, no. 6 (1976): 418–25.

Burleson, M. H., et al., "Heterosexual Activity and Cycle Length Variability: Effect of Gynecological Maturity," *Physiology and Behavior* 50 (1991): 863–66.

Catania, J. A., and C. B. White, "Sexuality in an Aged Sample: Cognitive Determinants of Masturbation," *Archives of Sexual Behavior* 11, no. 3 (1982): 237–45.

Charnetski, C. J., and F. X. Brennan, *Feeling Good Is Good for You: How Pleasure Can Boost Your Immune System and Lengthen Your Life* (Emmaus, Penn.: Rodale Press, 2001).

Coleman, E., "Masturbation as a Means of Achieving Sexual Health," *Journal of Psychology and Human Sexuality* 14, no. 2–3 (2002): 5–16.

Cutler, W. B., *Love Cycles: The Science of Intimacy* (New York: Villard Books, 1991).

Davey, S., et al., "Sex and Death: Are They Related? Findings from the Caerphilly Cohort Study," *British Medical Journal* 315 (1997): 1641–44.

Davies, S., et al., "Sexual Desire Discrepancies: Effects on Sexual and Relationship Satisfaction in Heterosexual Dating Couples," *Archives of Sexual Behavior* 28, no. 6 (1999): 553–67.

Ebrahim, S., et al., "Sexual Intercourse and Risk of Ischaemic Stroke and Coronary Heart Disease: The Caerphilly Study," *Journal of Epidemiology Community Health* 56 (2002): 99–102.

Ellison, C. R., *Women's Sexualities* (Oakland, Calif.: New Harbinger, 2000).

Evans, R. W., and J. R. Couch, "Orgasm and Migraine," *Headache* 41 (2001): 512–14.

Feldman, H. A., et al., "Low Dehydroepiandrosterone Sulfate and Heart Disease in Middle-Aged Men: Cross-Sectional Results from the Massachusetts Male Aging Study," *Annals of Epidemiology* 8, no. 4 (1998): 217–28.

Fisher, H. E., *The Sex Contract: The Evolution of Human Behavior* (New York: Quill, 1982).

Fisher, H. E., et al., "Defining the Brain Systems of Lust, Romantic Attraction, and Attachment," *Archives of Sexual Behavior* 31, no. 5 (2002): 413–19.

Hurlbert, D. F., and K. E. Whittaker, "The Role of Masturbation in Marital and Sexual Satisfaction: A Comparative Study of Female Masturbators and Non-masturbators," *Journal of Sex Education and Therapy* 17, no. 4 (1991): 272–82.

Janszky, J., et al., "Orgasmic Aura—A Report of Seven Cases," *Seizure* 13, no. 6 (September 2004): 441–44.

Janszky, J., et al., "Orgasmic Aura Originates from the Right Hemisphere," *Neurology* 58, no. 2 (January 22, 2002): 302–04.

Kaplan, H. S., "Desire—Why and How It Changes," *Redbook* 58 (October 1984); cited in Komisaruk and Whipple, "Suppression of Pain."

Keesling, B., *Rx Sex: Making Love Is the Best Medicine* (Alameda, Calif.: Hunter House, 2000).

Komisaruk, B. R., and B. Whipple, "The Suppression of Pain by Genital Stimulation in Females," *Annual Review of Sex Research* (1995): 151–86.

Lê, M. G., et al. "Characteristics of Reproductive Life and Risk of Breast Cancer in a Case-Control Study of Young Nulliparous Women," *Journal of Clinical Epidemiology* 42, no. 12 (1989): 1227–33.

Leitzmann, M. F., et al., "Ejaculation Frequency and Subsequent Risk of Prostate Cancer," *Journal of the American Medical Association* 291, no. 13 (April 7, 2004): 1578–86.

Levin, R. J., "The Physiology of Sexual Arousal in the Human Female: A Recreational and Progreational Synthesis," *Archives of Sexual Behavior* 31, no. 5 (2002): 405–11.

Manning, J., and R. Taylor, "Long Ring Fingers and Testosterone," *Evolution and Human Behavior* 22 (January 2001): 61–69.

Martin, S. M., J. T. Manning, and C. F. Dowrick, "Fluctuating Asymmetry, Relative Digit Length and Depression in Men," *Evolution and Human Behavior* 20 (1999): 203–14.

Meaddough, E. L., et al., "Sexual Activity, Orgasm and Tampon Use Are Associated with a Decreased Risk for Endometriosis," *Gynecologic and Obstetric Investigation* 53 (2002): 163–69.

Murrell, T. G. C., "The Potential for Oxytocin (OT) to Prevent Breast Cancer: A Hypothesis," *Breast Cancer Research and Treatment* 35 (1995): 225–29.

Odent, M., *The Scientification of Love* (London: Free Association Books, 1999).

Ogden, G., "Spiritual Passion and Compassion in Late-Life Sexual Relationships," *Electronic Journal of Human Sexuality* (August 14, 2001), http://www.ejhs.org/volume4/Ogden.htm.

Palmore, E., "Predictors of the Longevity Difference: A Twenty-Five Year Follow-Up," *Gerontologist* 22 (1982): 513–18.

Persson, G., "Five-Year Mortality in a 70-Year-Old Urban Population in Relation to Psychiatric Diagnosis, Personality, Sexuality and Early Parental Death," *Acta Psychiatrica Scandinavica* 64 (1981): 244–53.

Petridou, E., et al., "Endocrine Correlates of Male Breast Cancer Risk: A Case-Control Study in Athens, Greece," *British Journal of Cancer* 83, no. 9 (2000): 1234–37.

Sandel, M. E., et al., "Sexual Functioning Following Traumatic Brain Injury," *Brain Injury* 10, no. 10 (October 1996): 719–28.

Sayle, A. E., et al., "Sexual Activity During Late Pregnancy and Risk of Preterm Delivery," *Obstetrics and Gynecology* 97, no. 2 (2001): 283–89.

Shapiro, D., "Effect of Chronic Low Back Pain on Sexuality," *Medical Aspects of Human Sexuality* 17 (1983): 241–45; cited in Komisaruk and Whipple, "Suppressers of Pain."

Singh, D., et al., "Frequency and Timing of Coital Orgasm in Women Desirous of Becoming Pregnant," *Archives of Sexual Behavior* 27, no. 1 (1998): 15–29.

Spencer, N. A., et al., "Social Chemosignals from Breastfeeding Women Increase

Sexual Motivation," *Hormones and Behavior* 46, no. 3 (September 2004): 362–70.

Sprecher, S., "Sexual Satisfaction in Premarital Relationships: Associations with Satisfaction, Love, Commitment, and Stability," *Journal of Sex Research* 39, no. 3 (2002): 190–96.

Tur-Kaspa, I., et al., "How Often Should Infertile Men Have Intercourse to Achieve Conception?" *Fertility and Sterility* 62, no. 2 (1994): 370–75.

Von Sydow, K. "Sexuality During Pregnancy and After Childbirth: A Metacontent Analysis of 59 Studies," *Journal of Psychosomatic Research* 47, no. 1 (1999): 27–49.

Walters, A. S., and G. M. Williamson, "Sexual Satisfaction Predicts Quality of Life: A Study of Adult Amputees," *Sexuality and Disability* 16, no. 2 (1998): 103–15.

Warner, P., and J. Bancroft. "Mood, Sexuality, Oral Contraceptives and the Menstrual Cycle," *Journal of Psychosomatic Research* 32, nos. 4–5 (1988): 417–27.

Weeks, D., and J. James, *Secrets of the Superyoung* (New York: Berkley Books, 1998).

Whipple, B., and B. R. Komisaruk, "Elevation of Pain Threshold by Vaginal Stimulation in Women," *Pain* 21 (1985): 357–67.

Wilson, M., and M. Daly, "Do Pretty Women Inspire Men to Discount the Future?" *Proceedings of the Royal Society of London, Series B—Biological Sciences* 271, Suppl. 4 (May 7, 2004): S177–79.

Yavaşçaoğlu, İ., et al., "Role of Ejaculation in the Treatment of Chronic Non-Bacterial Prostatitis," *International Journal of Urology* 6 (1999): 130–34.

Zamboni, B. D., and I. Crawford, "Using Masturbation in Sex Therapy: Relationships Between Masturbation, Sexual Desire, and Sexual Fantasy," *Journal of Psychology and Human Sexuality* 14, nos. 2–3 (2002): 123–41.

CHAPTER 16

Baxter, L. R., Jr, et al., "Caudate Glucose Metabolic Rate Changes with Both Drug and Behavior Therapy for Obsessive-Compulsive Disorder," *Archives of General Psychiatry* 49, no. 9 (September 1992): 681–89.

Brody, A. L., et al., "FDG-PET Predictors of Response to Behavioral Therapy and Pharmacotherapy in Obsessive Compulsive Disorder," *Psychiatry Research* 84, no. 1 (November 9, 1998): 1–6.

Brody, A. L., et al., "Regional Brain Metabolic Changes in Patients with Major Depression Treated with Either Paroxetine or Interpersonal Therapy: Preliminary Findings," *Archives of General Psychiatry* 58, no. 7 (July 2001): 631–40.

Davidson, J. R., et al., "Fluoxetine, Comprehensive Cognitive Behavioral Therapy, and Placebo in Generalized Social Phobia," *Archives of General Psychiatry* 61, no. 10 (October 2004): 1005–13.

Findley, T., "The Placebo and the Physician," *Medical Clinics of North America* 1 (November 1983): 1821–26.

Frank, J. D., "The Dynamics of the Psychotherapeutic Relationship: Determinants and Effects of the Therapist's Influence," *Psychiatry* 22, no. 1 (February 1959): 17–39.

Furmark, T., et al., "Common Changes in Cerebral Blood Flow in Patients with Social Phobia Treated with Citalopram or Cognitive-Behavioral Therapy," *Archives of General Psychiatry* 59, no. 5 (May 2002): 425–33.

Goldapple, K., et al., "Modulation of Cortical-Limbic Pathways in Major Depression: Treatment-Specific Effects of Cognitive Behavior Therapy," *Archives of General Psychiatry* 61, no. 1 (January 2004): 34–41.

Levin, P., S. Lazrove, and B. van der Kolk, "What Psychological Testing and Neuroimaging Tell Us About the Treatment of Posttraumatic Stress Disorder by Eye Movement Desensitization and Reprocessing," *Journal of Anxiety Disorders* 13, nos. 1–2 (January–April 1999): 159–72.

Martin, S. D., et al., "Brain Blood Flow Changes in Depressed Patients Treated with Interpersonal Psychotherapy or Venlafaxine Hydrochloride: Preliminary Findings," *Archives of General Psychiatry* 58, no. 7 (July 2001): 641–48.

Nakatani, E., et al., "Effects of Behavior Therapy on Regional Cerebral Blood Flow in Obsessive-Compulsive Disorder," *Psychiatry Research* 124, no. 2 (October 30, 2003): 113–20.

Paquette, V., et al., " 'Change the Mind and You Change the Brain': Effects of Cognitive-Behavioral Therapy on the Neural Correlates of Spider Phobia," *Neuroimage* 18, no. 2 (February 2003): 401–09.

Prasko, J., et al., "The Change of Regional Brain Metabolism (18FDG PET) in Panic Disorder During the Treatment with Cognitive Behavioral Therapy or Antidepressants," *Neuroendocrinology Letters* 25, no. 5 (October 2004): 340–48.

Schwartz, J. M., et al., "Systematic Changes in Cerebral Glucose Metabolic Rate After Successful Behavior Modification Treatment of Obsessive-Compulsive Disorder," *Archives of General Psychiatry* 53, no. 2 (February 1996): 109–13.

CHAPTER 17

Bridgett, D. J., and J. Cuevas, "Effects of Listening to Mozart and Bach on the Performance of a Mathematical Test," *Perceptual and Motor Skills* 90 (2000): 1171–75.

Campbell, D., *The Mozart Effect: Tapping the Power of Music to Heal the Body, Strengthen the Mind, and Unlock the Creative Spirit* (New York: Avon, 1997).

Carlson, S., et al., "Effects of Music and White Noise on Working Memory Performance in Monkeys," *Neuroreport* 8 (1997): 2853–56.

Creutzfeldt, O., and G. Ojemann, "Neuronal Activity in the Human Lateral Temporal Lobe. III. Activity Changes During Music," *Experimental Brain Research* 77 (1989): 490–98.

Esch, T., et al., "Commonalities in the Central Nervous System's Involvement with Complementary Medical Therapies: Limbic Morphinergic Processes," *Medical Science Monitor* 10, no. 6 (June 2004): MS6–17.

Formisano, R., et al., "Active Music Therapy in the Rehabilitation of Severe Brain Injured Patients During Coma Recovery," *Annali dell'Istituto superiore di sanit'* 37, no. 4 (2001): 627–30.

Gruhn, W., N. Galley, and C. Kluth, "Do Mental Speed and Musical Abilities Interact?" *Annals of the New York Academy of Sciences* 999 (November 2003): 485–96.

Jausovec, N., and K. Habe, "The 'Mozart Effect': An Electroencephalographic Analysis Employing the Methods of Induced Event-Related Desynchronization/Synchronization and Event-Related Coherence," *Brain Topography* 16, no. 2 (Winter 2003): 73–84.

Johnson, J. K., et al., "Enhancement of Spatial-Temporal Reasoning After a Mozart Listening Condition in Alzheimer's Disease: A Case Study," unpublished.

Kim, W. S., et al., "Asymmetric Activation in the Prefrontal Cortex by Sound-Induced Affect," *Perceptual and Motor Skills* 97, no. 3, pt. 1 (December 2003): 847–54.

Koch, J. E., and F. R. Rauscher, "Development of Central Auditory and Spatial Processing Sites: The Effects of Exposure to Music," paper presented at the twenty-seventh annual meeting of the Society for Neuroscience, New Orleans, October 1997.

Miller, A., and D. Coen, "The Case for Music in the Schools," *Phi Delta Kappan* 75, no. 6: 459–61.

Pratt, R. R., "Art, Dance, and Music Therapy," *Physical Medicine and Rehabilitation Clinics of North America* 15, no. 4 (November 2004): 827–41, vi–viii.

Pratt, R. R., and D. E. Grocke, eds., *MusicMedicine*, vol. 3, *MusicMedicine and Music Therapy: Expanding Horizons* (MMB Music, 2001).

Rauscher, F. H., G. L. Shaw, and K. N. Ky, "Music and Spatial Task Performance," *Nature* 365 (1993): 611.

———, "Listening to Mozart Enhances Spatial-Temporal Reasoning: Towards a Neurophysiological Basis," *Neuroscience Letters* 185 (1995): 44–47.

Rauscher, F. H., et al., "Music Training Causes Long-Term Enhancement of Preschool Children's Spatial-Temporal Reasoning," *Neurological Research* 19 (1997): 2–8.

Rideout, B. E., and J. Taylor, "Enhanced Spatial Performance Following Ten Minutes Exposure to Music: A Replication," *Perceptual and Motor Skills* 85, no. 1 (August 1997): 112–14.

Shenoy, K. V., et al., "Learning by Selection in the Trion Model of Cortical Organization, *Cerebral Cortex* 3, no. 239 (1993): _____.

Sutoo, D., and K. Akiyama, "Music Improves Dopaminergic Neurotransmission: Demonstration Based on the Effect of Music on Blood Pressure Regulation," *Brain Research* 1016, no. 2 (August 6, 2004): 255–62.

CHAPTER 18

Berk, L. S., et al., "Modulation of Neuroimmune Parameters During the Eustress of Humor-Associated Mirthful Laughter," *Alternative Therapies in Health and Medicine* 7, no. 2 (March 2001): 62–72, 74–76.

Berk, L. S., et al., "Neuroendocrine and Stress Hormone Changes During Mirthful Laughter," *American Journal of Medical Science* 298, no. 6 (1989): 390–96.

Cousins, N., *Anatomy of an Illness As Perceived by the Patient* (New York: Bantam, 1991).

Dossey, L., *Healing Words* (San Francisco: HarperSanFrancisco, 1997).

Matthews, D. A., *Faith Factor* (New York: Penguin, 1999).

Murialdo, G., et al., "Relationships Between Cortisol, Dehydroepiandrosterone Sulphate and Insulin-like Growth Factor-I System in Dementia," *Journal of Endocrinological Investigation* 24 (2001): 139–46.

Newberg, A., *Why Won't God Go Away* (New York: Ballantine Books, 2003).

Sapolsky, R. M., *Why Zebras Don't Get Ulcers,* 3rd ed. (New York: Owl Books, 2004).

———, "Taming Stress," *Scientific American* 289, no. 3 (September 2003): 86–95.

———, "Depression, Antidepressants, and the Shrinking Hippocampus," *Proceedings of the National Academy of Science* 98, no. 22 (October 23, 2001): 12320–22.

CHAPTER 19

Bernhardt, T., K. Maurer, and L. Frolich, "Effect of Daily Living-Related Cognitive Training on Attention and Memory Performance of Persons with Dementia," *Zeitschrift für Gerontologic und Geriatric* 35 (2002): 32–38.

Bird, T. D., "Clinical Genetics of Familial Alzheimer's Disease," in R.D. Terry, et al., eds., *Alzheimer Disease* (Philadelphia: Lippincott Williams and Wilkins, 1999), 57–67.

Braak, E., et al., "Neuropathology of Alzheimer's Disease: What Is New Since A. Alzheimer?" *European Archives of Psychiatry and Clinical Neuroscience* 249 Suppl. 3 (1999): 14–22.

Broe, G. A., et al., "Health Habits and Risk of Cognitive Impairment and Dementia in Old Age: A Prospective Study on the Effects of Exercise, Smoking and Alcohol Consumption," *Australian and New Zealand Journal of Public Health* 22 (1998): 621–23.

Conquer, J. A., et al., "Fatty Acid Analysis of Blood Plasma of Patients with Alzheimer's Disease, Other Types of Dementia, and Cognitive Impairment," *Lipids* 35 (2000): 1305–12.

Corbo, R. M., and R. Scacchi, "Apolipoprotein E (APOE) Allele Distribution in the World. Is APOE*4 a 'Thrifty' Allele?" *Annals of Human Genetics* 63 (1999): 301–10.

Cotman, C. W., and N. C. Berchtold, "Exercise: A Behavioral Intervention to Enhance Brain Health and Plasticity," *Trends in Neuroscience* 25 (2002): 295–301.

Di Castelnuovo, A., et al., "Meta-Analysis of Wine and Beer Consumption in Relation to Vascular Risk," *Circulation* 105 (2002): 2836–44.

Engelhart, M. J., et al., "Dietary Intake of Antioxidants and Risk of Alzheimer Disease," *Journal of the American Medical Association* 287 (2002): 3261–63.

Eriksson, P. S., et al., "Neurogenesis in the Adult Human Hippocampus," *Nature Medicine* 4 (1998): 1313–17.

Farrag, A. K., et al., "Effect of Surgical Menopause on Cognitive Functions," *Dementia and Geriatric Cognitive Disorders* 13 (2002): 193–98.

Ficker, J. H., et al., "Changes in Regional CNS Perfusion in Obstructive Sleep Apnea Syndrome: Initial SPECT Studies with Injected Nocturnal 99mTc-HMPAO," *Pneumologie* 51 (1997): 926–30.

Kabuto, M., et al., "A Prospective Study of Estradiol and Breast Cancer in Japanese Women," *Cancer Epidemiology Biomarkers and Prevention* 9 (2000): 575–79.

Kalmijn, S., et al., "Metabolic Cardiovascular Syndrome and Risk of Dementia in Japanese-American Elderly Men. The Honolulu-Asia Aging Study," *Arteriosclerosis, Thrombosis, and Vascular Biology* 20 (2000): 2255–60.

Kawas, C., and R. Katzman, "Epidemiology of Dementia and Alzheimer's Disease," in R. D. Terry, et al., eds., *Alzheimer Disease* (Philadelphia: Lippincott Williams and Wilkins, 1999), 95–117.

Kawas, C., et al., "A Prospective Study of Estrogen Replacement Therapy and the Risk of Developing Alzheimer's Disease: The Baltimore Longitudinal Study of Aging," *Neurology* 48 (1997): 1517–21.

Kosunen, O., et al., "Relation of Coronary Atherosclerosis and Apolipoprotein E Genotypes in Alzheimer Patients," *Stroke* 26 (1995): 743–48.

Launer, L. J., et al., "The Association Between Midlife Blood Pressure Levels and Late-Life Cognitive Function. The Honolulu-Asia Aging Study," *Journal of the American Medical Association* 274 (1995): 1846–51.

Luchsinger, J. A., et al., "Caloric Intake and the Risk of Alzheimer Disease," *Archives of Neurology* 59 (2002): 1258–63.

McCleary, R., R. A. Mulnard, and W. R. Shankle, "Reproductive Health Risks in Dementia: Evidence from the 1986 National Mortality Followback Survey," *Alzheimer's Research* 2 (1996): 181–84.

Nelson, H. D., et al., "Postmenopausal Hormone Replacement Therapy: Scientific Review," *Journal of the American Medical Association* 288 (2002): 872–81.

Riley, K. P., et al., "Cognitive Function and Apolipoprotein E in Very Old Adults: Findings from the Nun Study," *Journal of Gerontology, Series B—Psychological Sciences and Social Sciences* 55, no. 2 (March 2000): S69–75.

Ruitenberg, A., et al., "Alcohol Consumption and Risk of Dementia: The Rotterdam Study," *Lancet* 359 (2002): 281–86.

Selkoe, D. J., "AD: Genotypes, Phenotype and Treatment," *Science* 275 (1997): 630–31.

Seshadri, S., et al., "Plasma Homocysteine as a Risk Factor for Dementia and Alzheimer's Disease," *New England Journal of Medicine* 346 (2002): 476–83.

Shankle, W. R., and D. G. Amen, *Preventing Alzheimer's: Ways to Prevent, Delay or Halt Alzheimer's and Other Forms of Memory Loss* (New York: Putnam, 2004).

Shankle, W. R., M. S. Rafii, and B. H. Landing, "Functional Relationships Associated with Pattern of Development in Developing Human Cerebral Cortex," *Concepts in Neuroscience* 4, no. 1 (1993): 77–87.

Shankle, W. R., et al., "Numbers of Neurons Per Column in the Developing Human Cerebral Cortex from Birth to 72 Months: Evidence for an Apparent Post-Natal Increase in Neuron Numbers," *Journal of Theoretical Biology* 191 (1998): 115–40.

Tang, M. X., et al., "Effect of Age, Ethnicity, and Head Injury on the Association Between APOE Genotypes and Alzheimer's Disease," *Annals of the New York Academy of Sciences* 802 (1996): 6–15.

Truelson, T., et al., "Amount and Type of Alcohol and Risk of Dementia: The Copenhagen City Heart Study," *Neurology* 59 (2002): 1313–19.

Valcour, V. G., et al., "The Detection of Dementia in the Primary Care Setting," *Archives of Internal Medicine* 160 (2000): 2964–68.

Van Kooten, F., et al., "The Dutch Vascular Factors in Dementia Study: Rationale and Design," *Journal of Neurology* 245 (1998): 32–39.

Van Dam, F. S., et al., "Impairment of Cognitive Function in Women Receiving Adjuvant Treatment for High-Risk Breast Cancer: High-Dose Versus Standard-Dose Chemotherapy," *Journal of the National Cancer Institute* 90 (1998): 210–18.

Wilson, R. S., et al., "Participation in Cognitively Stimulating Activities and Risk of Incident Alzheimer Disease," *Journal of the American Medical Association* 287 (2002): 742–48.

Wilson, R. S., et al., "The Apolipoprotein E Varepsilon 2 Allele and Decline in Episodic Memory," *Journal of Neurology, Neurosurgery, and Psychiatry* 73 (2002): 672–77.

Yaffe, K., et al., "Estrogen Receptor 1 Polymorphisms and Risk of Cognitive Impairment in Older Women," *Biological Psychiatry* 51 (2002): 677–82.

CHAPTER 20

Acetyl-L-Carnitine

Brooks, J. O., III, et al., "Acetyl-L-Carnitine Slows Decline in Younger Patients with Alzheimer's Disease: A Reanalysis of a Double-Blind, Placebo-Controlled Trial Using the Trilinear Approach," *International Psychogeriatrics* 10 (1998): 193–203.

Cipolli, C., and G. Chiari, "Effects of L-Acetyl Carnitine on Mental Deterioration in the Aged: Initial Results," *Clinical Therapeutics* 132 (1990): 479–510.

Garzya, G., et al., "Evaluation of the Effects of L-Acetyl Carnitine on Senile Patients Suffering from Depression," *Drugs Under Experimental and Clinical Research* 16 (1990): 101–06.

Gorini, A., A. D'Angelo, and R. F. Villa, "Action of L-Acetylcarnitine on Different Cerebral Mitochondrial Populations from Cerebral Cortex," *Neurochemical Research* 23 (1998): 1485–91.

Guarnaschelli, C., G. Fugassa, and C. Pistarini, "Pathological Brain Ageing: Evaluation of the Efficacy of a Pharmacological Aid," *Drugs Under Experimental and Clinical Research* 14 (1998): 715–18.

Lolic, M. M., G. Fiskum, and R. E. Rosenthal, "Neuroprotective Effects of Acetyl-L-Carnitine After Stroke in Rats," *Annals of Emergency Medicine* 29 (1997): 758–65.

Patti, F., P. Marano, and S. Cappello, "Effects of L-Acetyl Carnitine on Functional Recovery of Hemiplegic Patients," *Clinical Trials Journal* 25 (1988): 87–101.

Pettegrew, J. W., W. E. Klunke, and K. Panchalingam, "Clinical and Biochemical Effects of Acetyl-L-Carnitine in Alzheimer's Disease," *Neurobiology of Aging* 16 (1998): 1–4.

Rai, G., et al., "Double-Blind, Placebo-Controlled Study of Acetyl-l-Carnitine in Patients with Alzheimer's Dementia," *Current Medical Research and Opinion* 11 (1990): 638–47.

Salvioli, G., and M. Neri, "L-Acetylcarnitine Treatment of Mental Decline in the Elderly," *Drugs Under Experimental and Clinical Research* 20 (1994): 169–76.

Sano, M., et al., "Double-Blind Parallel Pilot Study of Acetyl Levocarnitine in Patients with Alzheimer's Disease," *Archives of Neurology* 49 (1992): 1137–41.

Spagnoli, A., et al., "Long-Term Acetyl-L-Carnitine Treatment in Alzheimer's Disease," *Neurology* 41 (1991): 1726–32.

Tempesta, E., et al., "Role of Acetyl-L-Carnitine in the Treatment of Cognitive Deficit in Chronic Alcoholism," *International Journal of Clinical Pharmacological Research* 10 (1990): 101–07.

Tempesta, E., et al., "L-Acetylcarnitine in Depressed Elderly Subjects. A Cross-over Study vs. Placebo," *Drugs Under Experimental and Clinical Research* 10 (1990): 101–07.

Thal, L. J., et al., "A One Year Multicenter Placebo-Controlled Study of Acetyl-L-Carnitine in Patients with Alzheimer's Disease," *Neurology* 47 (1996): 705–11.

Alpha-Lipoic Acid

Marangon, K., et al., "Comparison of the Effect of Alpha-Lipoic Acid and Alpha-Tocopherol Supplementation on Measures of Oxidative Stress," *Free Radical Biology and Medicine* 27 (1999): 1114–21.

Packer, L., H. J. Tritschler, and K. Wessel, "Neuroprotection by the Metabolic Antioxidant Alpha-Lipoic Acid," *Free Radical Biology and Medicine* 22 (1997): 359–78.

Packer, L., E. H. Witt, and H. J. Tritschler, "Alpha-Lipoic as a Biological Antioxidant," *Free Radical Biology and Medicine* 79 (1995): 227–50.

Poon, H. F., et al., "Proteomic Analysis of Specific Brain Proteins in Aged SAMP8 Mice Treated with Alpha-Lipoic Acid: Implications for Aging and Age-Related Neurodegenerative Disorders," *Neurochemistry International* 46, no. 2 (January 2005): 159–68.

Tirosh, O., et al., "Neuroprotective Effects of Alpha-Lipoic Acid and Its Positively Charged Amide Analogue," *Free Radical Biology and Medicine* 26 (1999): 1418–26.

Ziegler, D., et al., "Treatment of Symptomatic Diabetic Peripheral Neuropathy with the Antioxidant Alpha-Lipoic Acid. A Three-Week Multicentre Randomized Controlled Trial (ALADIN Study)," *Diabetologia* 38 (1995): 1425–33.

CoQ10

Baggio, E., et al., "Italian Multicenter Study on the Safety and Efficacy of Coenzyme Q_{10} as Adjunctive Therapy in Heart Failure," *Molecular Aspects of Medicine* 15 (Suppl.) (1994): 287–94.

Chopra, R. K., et al., "Relative Bioavailability of Coenzyme Q_{10} Formulations in Human Subjects," *International Journal for Vitamin and Nutrition Research* 68 (1998): 109–13.

Crane, F. L., I. L. Sun, and E. E. Sun, "The Essential Functions of Coenzyme Q," *Clinical Investigator* 71 (Suppl.) (1993): S55–59.

Folkers, K., et al., "Lovastatin Decreases Coenzyme Q Levels in Humans," *Proceedings of the National Academy of Science* 87 (1990): 8931–34.

Hanaki, Y., et al., "Coenzyme Q_{10} and Coronary Artery Disease," *Clinical Investigator* 71 (Suppl.) (1993): S112–15.

Matthews, R. T., et al., "Coenzyme Q_{10} Administration Increases Mitochondrial Concentrations and Exerts Neuroprotective Effects," *Proceedings of the National Academy of Science* 95 (1998): 8892–97.

Shults, C. W., et al., "Pilot Trial of High Dosages of Coenzyme Q10 in Patients with Parkinson's Disease," *Experimental Neurology* 188, no. 2 (August 2004): 491–94.

Spigset, O., "Reduced Effect of Warfarin Caused by Ubidecarenone," *Lancet* 344 (1994): 1372–73.

Fish Oil

Adler, A. J., and B. J. Holub, "Effect of Garlic and Fish-Oil Supplementation on Serum Lipid and Lipoprotein Concentrations in Hypercholesterolemic Men," *American Journal of Clinical Nutrition* 65 (1997): 445–50.

Appel, L. J., et al., "Does Supplementation of Diet with 'Fish Oil' Reduce Blood Pressure? A Meta-Analysis of Controlled Clinical Trials," *Archives of Internal Medicine* 153 (1993): 1429–38.

Ariza-Ariza, R., M. Mestanza-Peralta, and M. H. Cardiel, "Omega-3 Fatty Acid in Rheumatoid Arthritis: An Overview," *Seminars in Arthritis and Rheumatism* 27 (1998): 366–70.

Belluzi, A., et al., "Effect of an Enteric-Coated Fish-Oil Preparation on Relapses in Crohn's Disease," *New England Journal of Medicine* 334 (1996): 1557–60.

GISSI-Prevenzione Investigators, "Dietary Supplementation with N-3 Polyunsaturated Fatty Acids and Vitamin E After Myocardial Infarction: Results of the GISSI-Prevenzione Trial," *Lancet* 354 (1999): 447–55.

Grimsgaard, S., et al., "Highly Purified Eicosapentaenoic Acid and Docosahexaenoic Acids in Humans Have Similar Triacylglycerol-Lowering Effects but Divergent Effects on Serum Fatty Acids," *American Journal of Clinical Nutrition* 66 (1997): 649–59.

Saldeen, P., and T. Saldeen, "Women and Omega-3 Fatty Acids," *Obstetrical and Gynecological Survey* 59, no. 10 (October 2004): 722–30, 745–46.

Stoll, A. L., et al., "Omega-3 Fatty Acids in Bipolar Disorder," *Archives of General Psychiatry* 56 (1999): 407–12.

Ginkgo Biloba

Blume, J., M. Kieser, and U. Holscher, "[Placebo-Controlled Double-Blind Study of the Effectiveness of Ginkgo Biloba Special Extract EGb 761 in Trained Patients with Intermittent Claudication]," *Vasa* 25, no. 3 (1996): 265–74.

———, [Ginkgo-Special-Extract EGb 761 in Peripheral Arterial Occlusive Diseases Stage IIb According to Fontaine], *Fortschritte Jer Medizin* 116, nos. 35–36 (1998): 36–37.

Blumenthal, M., A. Goldberg, J. Brinckmann, eds; Tyler, V. E., *Herbal Medicine: Expanded Commission E Monographs* (American Botanical Council, 2000).

Blumenthal, M., et al., eds, Klein, S.; R. S. Rister, trans, V. E. Tyler, *The Complete German Commission E Monographs: Therapeutic Guide to Herbal Medicines* (American Botanical Council, 1998).

Haase, J., P. Halama, and R. Horr, "Effectiveness of Brief Infusions with Ginkgo Biloba Special Extract EGb 761 in Dementia of the Vascular and Alzheimer Type," *Zeitschrift für Gerontologic und Geriatric* 29, no. 4 (1996): 302–09.

Hofferberth, B., "The Effect of Ginkgo Biloba Extract on Neurophysiological and Psychometric Measurement Results in Patients with Psychotic Organic Brain Syndrome. A Double-Blind Study Against Placebo," *Arzneimittelforschung* 39, no. 8 (1989): 918–22.

Kanowski, S., et al., "Proof of the Efficacy of the Ginkgo Biloba Special Extract EGb 761 in Outpatients Suffering from Mild to Moderate Primary Degenerative Dementia of the Alzheimer Type of Multi-Infarct Dementia," *Phytomedicine* 4 (1997): 3–13.

Kennedy, D. O., A. B. Scholey, and K. A. Wesnes, "The Dose-Dependent Cognitive Effects of Acute Administration of Ginkgo Biloba to Healthy Young Volunteers," *Psychopharmacology* 151, no. 4 (2000): 416–23.

Le Bars, P. L., et al., "A Placebo-Controlled, Double-Blind, Randomized Trial of an Extract of Ginkgo Biloba for Dementia. North American EGb Study Group," *Journal of the American Medical Association* 278, no. 16 (1997): 1327–32.

Le Bars, P. L., M. Kieser, and K. Z. Itil, "A 26-Week Analysis of a Double-Blind, Placebo-Controlled Trial of the Ginkgo Biloba Extract EGb 761 in Dementia," *Dementia and Geriatric Cognitive Disorders* 11, no. 4 (2000): 230–37.

Mix, J. A., and W. D. Crews, Jr., "An Examination of the Efficacy of Ginkgo Biloba Extract EGb 761 on the Neuropsychologic Functioning of Cognitively Intact Older Adults," *Journal of Alternative and Complementary Medicine* 6, no. 3 (2000): 219–29.

Oken, B. S., D. M. Storzbach, and J. A. Kaye, "The Efficacy of Ginkgo Biloba on Cognitive Function in Alzheimer Disease," *Archives of Neurology* 55, no. 11 (1998): 1409–15.

Rigney, U., S. Kimber, and I. Hindmarch, "The Effects of Acute Doses of Standardized Ginkgo Biloba Extract on Memory and Psychomotor Performance in Volunteers," *Phytotherapy Research* 13, no. 5 (1999): 408–15.

Santos, R. F., et al., "Cognitive Performance, SPECT, and Blood Viscosity in Elderly Non-Demented People Using Ginkgo Biloba," *Pharmacopsychiatry* 36, no. 4 (July 2003): 127–33.

Stough, C., et al., "Neuropsychological Changes After 30-Day Ginkgo Biloba Administration in Healthy Participants," *International Journal of Neuropsychopharmacology* 4, no. 2 (2001): 131–34.

Wesnes, K. A., et al., "The Memory Enhancing Effects of a Ginkgo Biloba/Panax Ginseng Combination in Healthy Middle-aged Volunteers," *Psychopharmacology* 152, no. 4 (2000): 353–61.

Yoshikawa, T., Y. Naito, and M. Kondo, "Ginkgo Biloba Leaf Extract: Review of Biological Actions and Clinical Applications," *Antioxidants and Redox Signaling* 1, no. 4 (1999): 469–80.

Phosphatidylserine

Amaducc, L., and SMID Group, "Phosphatidylserine in the Treatment of Alzheimer's Disease. Results of a Multicenter Study," *Psychopharmacology Bulletin* 24 (1988): 130–34.

Crook, T., et al., "Effects of Phosphatidylserine in Alzheimer's Disease," *Psychopharmacology Bulletin* 28 (1992): 61–66.

Crook, T. H., et al., "Effects of Phosphatidylserine in Age-Associated Memory Impairment," *Neurology* 41 (1991): 644–49.

Pepeu, G., I., Marconcini Pepeu, and L. Amaducc, "A Review of Phosphatidylserine Pharmacological and Clinical Effects. Is Phosphatidylserine a Drug for the Ageing Brain?" *Pharmacological Research* 33 (1996): 73–80.

Villardita, C., et al., "Multicentre Clinical Trial of Brain Phophatidylserine in Elderly Patients with Intellectual Deterioration," *Clinical Trials Journal* 24 (1987): 84–93.

Zanott, A., L. Valzelli, and G. Toffano, "Chronic Phosphatidylserine Treatment Improves Spatial Memory and Passive Avoidance in Aged Rats," *Psychopharmacology* 99 (1989): 316–21.

L-Theanine

Juneja, L. R., et al., "L-Theanine—A Unique Amino Acid of Green Tea and Its Relaxation Effect in Humans," *Trends in Food Science and Technology* 10 (1999): 199–204.

Lu, K., et al., "The Acute Effects of L-Theanine in Comparison with Alprazolam on Anticipatory Anxiety in Humans," *Human Psychopharmacology* 19, no. 7 (October 2004): 457–65.

Sadzuka, Y., et al., "The Effects of Theanine, as a Novel Biochemical Modulator, on the Antitumor Activity of Adriamycin," *Cancer Letters* 105 (1996): 203–09.

Vinpocetine

Bereczki, D., and I. Fekete, "A Systematic Review of Vinpocetine Therapy in Acute Ischaemic Stroke," *European Journal of Clinical Pharmacology* 55 (1999): 349–52.

Gulyas, B., et al., "Brain Uptake and Plasma Metabolism of [11C] Vinpocetine: A Preliminary PET Study in a Cynomolgus Monkey," *Journal of Neuroimaging* 9 (1999): 217–22.

Sitges, M., and V. Nekrassov, "Vinpocetine Prevents 4-Aminopyridine-Induced Changes in the EEG, the Auditory Brainstem Responses and Hearing," *Clinical Neurophysiology* 115, no. 12 (December 2004): 2711–17.

Thal, L. J., et al., "The Safety and Lack of Efficacy of Vinpocetine in Alzheimer's Disease," *Journal of the American Geriatrics Society* 37 (1989): 515–20.

Multiple Vitamins

Fletcher, R. H., and K. M. Fairfield, "Vitamins for Chronic Disease Prevention in Adults: Clinical Applications," *Journal of the American Medical Association* 287, no. 23 (June 19, 2002): 3127–29.

Vitamin B

Aarsand, A. K., and S. M. Carlsen, "Folate Administration Reduces Circulating Homocysteine Levels in NIDDM Patients on Long-term Metformin Treatment," *Journal of Internal Medicine* 244 (1998): 169–74.

Anon., "How Folate Fights Disease," *Nature Structural Biology* 6 (1999): 293–94.

Baik, H. W., and R. M. Russell, "Vitamin B_{12} Deficiency in the Elderly," *Annual Review of Nutrition* 19 (1999): 357–77.

Berry, R. J., et al., "Prevention of Neural-Tube Defects with Folic Acid in China," *New England Journal of Medicine* 341 (1999): 1485–90.

Bottiglieri, T., "Folate, Vitamin B_{12}, and Neuropsychiatric Disorders," *Nutrition Reviews* 54 (1996): 382–90.

Boushey, C. J., et al., "A Quantitative Assessment of Plasma Homocysteine as a Risk Factor for Vascular Disease. Probable Benefits of Increasing Folic Acid Intakes," *Journal of the American Medical Association* 274 (1995): 1049–57.

Clarke, R., et al., "Folate, Vitamin B_{12}, and Serum Total Homocysteine Levels in Confirmed Alzheimer's Disease," *Archives of Neurology* 55 (1998): 1449–55.

Coppen, A., and J. Bailey, "Enhancement of the Antidepressant Action of Fluoxetine by Folic Acid: A Randomized, Placebo-Controlled Trial," *Journal of Affective Disorders* 60 (2000): 121–30.

Coppen, A., S. Chaudhry, and C. Swade, "Folic Acid Enhances Lithium Prophylaxis," *Journal of Affective Disorders* 10 (1986): 9–13.

Czeizel, A. E., and I. Dudás, "Prevention of the First Occurrence of Neural-Tube Defects by Periconceptional Vitamin Supplementation," *New England Journal of Medicine* 327 (1992): 1832–35.

Guilarte, T. R., "Vitamin B_6 and Cognitive Development: Recent Research Findings from Human and Animal Studies," *Nutrition Reviews* 51 (1993): 193–98.

Homocysteine Lowering Trialists' Collaboration, "Lowering Blood Homocysteine with Folic Acid Based Supplements: Meta-Analysis of Randomized Trials," *British Medical Journal* 316 (1998): 894–98.

Leklem, J. E., "Vitamin B_6," in M.E. Shils et al., eds, *Modern Nutrition in Health and Disease*, 9th ed. (Baltimore: Williams and Wilkins, 1999), 413–21.

Lindenbaum, J., et al., "Neuropsychiatric Disorders Caused by Cobalamin Deficiency in the Absence of Anemia or Macrocytosis," *New England Journal of Medicine* 318 (1988): 1720–28.

McCaddon, A., and C. L. Kelly, "Familial Alzheimer's Disease and Vitamin B_{12} Deficiency," *Age and Ageing* 23 (1994): 334–37.

Rimm, E. B., et al., "Higher Intake of Folate and Vitamin B_6 Is Associated with Low Rates of Coronary Artery Disease in Women," *Journal of the American Medical Association* 279 (1998): 359–64.

Snowdon, D. A., et al., "Serum Folate and the Severity of Atrophy of the Neocortex in Alzheimer Disease: Findings from the Nun Study," *American Journal of Clinical Nutrition* 71 (2000): 993–98.

Sumner, A. E., et al., "Elevated Methylmalonic Acid and Total Homocysteine Levels Show High Prevalence of Vitamin B_{12} Deficiency After Gastric Surgery," *Annals of Internal Medicine* 124 (1996): 469–76.

Weir, D. G., and J. M. Scott, "Brain Function in the Elderly: Role of Vitamin B_{12} and Folate," *British Medical Bulletin* 55 (1999): 669–82.

Wyatt, K. M., et al., "Efficacy of Vitamin B_6 in the Treatment of Premenstrual Syndrome: Systemic Review," *British Medical Journal* 318 (1999): 1375–81.

Vitamin C

Age-Related Eye Disease Study Research Group, "A Randomized, Placebo-Controlled, Clinical Trial of High-Dose Supplementation with Vitamins C and E, Beta Carotene, and Zinc for Age-Related Macular Degeneration and Vision Loss: AREDS Report No. 8," *Archives of Ophthalmology* 119, no. 10 (October 2001): 1417–36.

Dietary Reference Intakes for Vitamin C, Vitamin E, Selenium, and Carotenoids (Washington, D.C.: National Academy Press, 2000).

Engelhart, M. J., et al., "Dietary Intake of Antioxidants and Risk of Alzheimer Disease," *Journal of the American Medical Association* 287, no. 24 (June 26, 2002): 3223–29.

Gray, S. L., et al., "Is Antioxidant Use Protective of Cognitive Function in the Community-Dwelling Elderly?" *American Journal of Geriatric Pharmacotherapy* 1, no. 1 (September 2003): 3–10.

Lykkesfeldt, J., et al., "Ascorbate Is Depleted by Smoking and Repleted By Moderate Supplementation: A Study in Male Smokers and Nonsmokers with Matched Dietary Intakes," *American Journal of Clinical Nutrition* 71 (2000): 530–36.

Voko, Z., et al., "Dietary Antioxidants and the Risk of Ischemic Stroke: The Rotterdam Study," *Neurology* 61, no. 9 (November 11, 2003): 1273–75.

Vitamin E

Adler, L. A., et al., "Vitamin E Treatment for Tardive Dyskinesia," *Archives of General Psychiatry* 56 (1999): 836–41.

Anderson, D. K., T. R. Waters, and E. D. Means, "Pretreatment with Alpha-Tocopherol Enhances Neurologic Recovery After Experimental Spinal Cord Compression Injury," *Journal of Neurotrauma* 5, no. 61 (1998): 61–67.

Aslam, A., et al., "Vitamin E Deficiency Induced Neurological Disease in Common Variable Immunodeficiency: Two Cases and a Review of the Literature of Vitamin E Deficiency," *Clinical Immunology* 112, no. 1 (July 2004): 24–29.

Engelhart, M. J., et al., "Dietary Intake of Antioxidants and Risk of Alzheimer Disease," *Journal of the American Medical Association* 287, no. 24 (June 26, 2002): 3223–29.

GISSI-Prevenzione Investigators, "Dietary Supplementation with N-3 Polyunsaturated Fatty Acids and Vitamin E after Myocardial Infarction: Results of the GISSI-Prevenzioni Trial," *Lancet* 354 (1999): 447–55.

Gray, S. L., et al., "Predictors of Nutritional Supplement Use by the Elderly," *Pharmacotherapy* 16, no. 4 (July–August 1996): 715–20.

Gray, S. L., et al., "Is Antioxidant Use Protective of Cognitive Function in the Community-Dwelling Elderly?" *American Journal of Geriatric Pharmacotherapy* 1, no. 1 (September 2003): 3–10.

Grundman, M., "Vitamin E and Alzheimer's Disease: The Basis for Additional Clinical Trials," *American Journal of Clinical Nutrition* 71 (2000): 630S–36S.

Miller, E. R., III, et al., "Meta-Analysis: High-Dosage Vitamin E Supplementation May Increase All-Cause Mortality," *Annals of Internal Medicine* (January 4, 2005): 37–46.

Rimm, E. B., et al., "Vitamin E Consumption and the Risk of Coronary Heart Disease in Men," *New England Journal of Medicine* 328, no. 20 (May 20, 1993): 1450–56.

Rutten, B. P., et al., "Antioxidants and Alzheimer's Disease: From Bench to Bedside (and Back Again)," *Current Opinion in Clinical Nutrition and Metabolic Care* 5, no. 6 (November 2002): 645–51.

Shoulson, I., "DATATOP: A Decade of Neuroprotective Inquiry. Parkinson Study Group. Deprenyl and Tocopherol Antioxidative Therapy of Parkinsonism," *Annals of Neurology* 44, no. 3 suppl. 1 (1998): S160–66.

Stampfer, M. J., et al., "Vitamin E Consumption and the Risk of Coronary Disease in Women," *New England Journal of Medicine* 328, no. 20 (May 20, 1993): 1444–49.

Traber, M. G., "Which Form of Vitamin E, Alpha- or Gamma-Tocopherol, Is Better?" Linus Pauling Institute Report (2002).

Voko, Z., et al., "Dietary Antioxidants and the Risk of Ischemic Stroke: The Rotterdam Study," *Neurology* 61, no. 9 (November 11, 2003): 1273–75.

Wu, A., Z. Ying, and F. Gomez-Pinilla, "The Interplay Between Oxidative Stress and Brain-Derived Neurotrophic Factor Modulates the Outcome of a Saturated Fat Diet on Synaptic Plasticity and Cognition," *European Journal of Neuroscience* 19, no. 7 (April 2004): 1699–707.

SAMe

Bell, K. M., et al., "S-Adenosylmethionine Treatment of Depression: A Controlled Clinical Trial," *American Journal of Psychiatry* 145, no. 9 (1988): 1110–14.

Bell, K. M., et al., "S-Adenosylmethionine Blood Levels in Major Depression: Changes with Drug Treatment," *Acta Neurologica Scandinavica* 154 (Suppl.) (1994): 15–18.

Berlanga, C., et al., "Efficacy of S-Adenosyl-L-Methionine in Speeding the Onset of Action of Imipramine," *Psychiatry Research* 44, no. 3 (1992): 257–62.

Glorioso, S., et al., "Double-Blind Multicentre Study of the Activity of S-Adenosylmethionine in Hip and Knee Osteoarthritis," *International Journal of Clinical Pharmacology Research* 5, no. 1 (1985): 39–49.

Jacobsen, S., B. Danneskiold-Samsoe, and R. B. Andersen, "Oral S-Adenosylmethionine in Primary Fibromyalgia. Double-Blind Clinical Evaluation," *Scandinavian Journal of Rheumatology* 20, no. 4 (1991): 294–302.

Kagan, B. L., et al., "Oral S-Adenosylmethionine in Depression: A Randomized, Double-Blind, Placebo-Controlled Trial," *American Journal of Psychiatry* 147, no. 5 (1990): 591–95.

Maccagno, A., et al., "Double-Blind Controlled Clinical Trial of Oral S-Adenosylmethionine Versus Piroxicam in Knee Osteoarthritis," *American Journal of Medicine* 83, no. 5A (1987): 72–77.

Mantero, M., et al., "Controlled Double-Blind Study (SAMe-Imipramine) in Depressive Syndromes," *Minerva Medica* 66, no. 78 (1975): 4098–101.

Muller-Fassbender, H., "Double-Blind Clinical Trial of S-Adenosylmethionine Versus Ibuprofen in the Treatment of Osteoarthritis," *American Journal of Medicine* 83, no. 5A (1987): 81–83.

Salmaggi, P., et al., "Double-Blind, Placebo-Controlled Study of S-Adenosyl-L-Methionine in Depressed Postmenopausal Women," *Psychotherapy and Psychosomatics* 59, no. 1 (1993): 34–40.

Tavoni, A., et al., "Evaluation of S-Adenosylmethionine in Primary Fibromyalgia. A Double-Blind Crossover Study," *American Journal of Medicine* 83, no. 5A (1987): 107–10.

Vetter, G., "Double-Blind Comparative Clinical Trial with S-Adenosylmethionine and Indomethacin in the Treatment of Osteoarthritis," *American Journal of Medicine* 83, no. 5A (1987): 78–80.

Volkmann, H., et al., "Double-Blind, Placebo-Controlled Cross-over Study of Intravenous S-Adenosyl-L-Methionine in Patients with Fibromyalgia," *Scandinavian Journal of Rheumatology* 26, no. 3 (1997): 206–11.

St. John's Wort

Behnke, K., et al., "Hypericum Perforatum Versus Fluoxetine in the Treatment of Mild to Moderate Depression," *Advances in Therapy* 19, no. 1 (2002): 43–52.

Brenner, R., et al., "Comparison of an Extract of Hypericum (LI 160) and Sertraline in the Treatment of Depression: A Double-blind, Randomized Pilot Study," *Clinical Therapeutics* 22, no. 4 (2000): 411–19.

Czekalla, J., et al., "The Effect of Hypericum Extract on Cardiac Conduction as Seen in the Electrocardiogram Compared to that of Imipramine," *Pharmacopsychiatry* 30, suppl. 2 (1990): 86–88.

Friede, M., H. H. Henneicke von Zepelin, and J. Freudenstein, "Differential Therapy of Mild to Moderate Depressive Episodes (ICD-10 F 32.0; F 32.1) with St. John's Wort," *Pharmacopsychiatry* 34, Suppl 1 (2001): S38–41.

Hansgen, K., D. J. Vesper, and M. Ploch, "Multicenter Double-Blind Study Examining the Antidepressant Effectiveness of the Hypericum Extract LI 160," *Journal of Geriatric Psychiatry and Neurology* 7, Suppl. 1 (1994): S15–18.

Harrer, G., W. D. Hubner, and H. Podzuweit, "Effectiveness and Tolerance of the Hypericum Extract LI 160 Compared to Maprotiline: A Multicenter Double-Blind Study," *Journal of Geriatric Psychiatry and Neurology* 7, Suppl. 1 (1994): S24–28.

Hubner, W. D., S. Lande, and H. Podzuweit, "Hypericum Treatment of Mild Depressions with Somatic Symptoms," *Journal of Geriatric Psychiatry and Neurology* 7, Suppl. 1 (1994): S12–14.

Johnson, D., et al., "Effects of Hypericum Extract LI 160 Compared with Maprotiline on Resting EEG and Evoked Potentials in 24 Volunteers," *Journal of Geriatric Psychiatry and Neurology* 7, Suppl. 1 (1994): S44–46.

Kalb, R., R. D. Trautmann-Sponsel, and M. Kieser, "Efficacy and Tolerability of Hypericum Extract WS 5572 Versus Placebo in Mildly to Moderately Depressed Patients. A Randomized Double-Blind Multicenter Clinical Trial," *Pharmacopsychiatry* 34, no. 3 (2001): 96–103.

Laakmann, G., et al., "St. John's Wort in Mild to Moderate Depression: The Relevance of Hyperforin for the Clinical Efficacy," *Pharmacopsychiatry* 31, Suppl 1 (1998): 54–59.

Philipp, M., R. Kohnen, and K. O. Hiller, "Hypericum Extract Versus Imipramine or Placebo in Patients with Moderate Depression: Randomised Multicentre Study of Treatment for Eight Weeks," *British Medical Journal* 319, no. 7224 (1999): 1534–38.

Sommer, H., and G. Harrer, "Placebo-Controlled Double-Blind Study Examining the Effectiveness of an Hypericum Preparation in 105 Mildly Depressed Patients," *Journal of Geriatric Psychiatry and Neurology* 7, Suppl 1 (1994): S9–11.

Witte, B., et al., "Treatment of Depressive Symptoms with a High Concentration

Hypericum Preparation. A Multicenter Placebo-Controlled Double-Blind Study," *Fortschrilt der Medizin* 113, no. 28 (1995): 404–08.

Vorbach, E. U., W. D. Hubner, and K. H. Arnoldt, "Effectiveness and Tolerance of the Hypericum Extract LI 160 in Comparison with Imipramine: Randomized Double-Blind Study with 135 Outpatients," *Journal of Geriatric Psychiatry and Neurology* 7, Suppl. 1 (1994): S19–23.

5-HTP

Alino, J. J., L. Gutierrez, and M. L. Iglesias, "5-Hydroxytryptophan (5-HTP) and a MAOI (Nialamide) in the Treatment of Depressions. A Double-Blind Controlled Study," *International Pharmacopsychiatry* 11, no. 1 (1976): 8–15.

Kahn, R. S., et al., "Effect of a Serotonin Precursor and Uptake Inhibitor in Anxiety Disorders: A Double-Blind Comparison of 5-Hydroxytryptophan, Clomipramine and Placebo," *International Clinical Psychopharmacology* 2, no. 1 (1987): 33–45.

Nardini, M., et al., "Treatment of Depression with L-5-Hydroxytryptophan Combined with Chloɪimipramine, A Double-Blind Study," *International Journal of Clinical Pharmacology Research* 3, no. 4 (1983): 239–50.

Ribeiro, C. A., "L-5-hydroxytryptophan in the Prophylaxis of Chronic Tension-type Headache: A Double-Blind, Randomized, Placebo-Controlled Study. For the Portuguese Head Society," *Headache* 40, no. 6 (2000): 451–56.

Rousseau, J. J., "Effects of a Levo-5-Hydroxytryptophan-Dihydroergocristine Combination on Depression and Neuropsychic Performance: A Double-Blind Placebo-Controlled Clinical Trial in Elderly Patients," *Clinical Therapeutics* 9, no. 3 (1987): 267–72.

Inositol

Barak, Y., et al., "Inositol Treatment of Alzheimer's Disease: A Double-Blind, Cross-over Placebo-Controlled Trial," *Progress in Neuro-psychopharmacological and Biological Psychiatry* 20 (1996): 729–35.

Benjamin, J., et al., "Double-Blind, Placebo-Controlled, Crossover Trial of Inositol Treatment for Panic Disorder," *American Journal of Psychiatry* 152 (1995): 1084–86.

Einat, H., et al., "Inositol Reduces Depressive-like Behaviors in Two Different Models of Depression," *Psychopharmacology* 144 (1999): 158–62.

Fox, M., et al., "Inositol Treatment of Obsessive-Compulsive Disorder," *American Journal of Psychiatry* 153 (1996): 1219–21.

Levine, J., "Controlled Trials of Inositol in Psychiatry," *European Neuropsychopharmacology* 7 (1997): 147–55.

Levine, J., et al., "Double-Blind, Controlled-Trial of Inositol Treatment of Depression," *American Journal of Psychiatry* 152 (1995): 792–94.

Levine, J., et al., "CSF Inositol in Schizophrenia and High-Dose Inositol Treatment of Schizophrenic," *European Neuropsychopharmacology* 4 (1994): 487–90.

Seedat, S., and D. J. Stein, "Inositol Augmentation of Serotonin Reuptake Inhibitors in Treatment-Refractory Obsessive-Compulsive Disorder: An Open Trial," *International Clinical Psychopharmacology* 14 (1999): 353–56.

Valerian

Davidson, J. R. T., and K. M. Connor, "Valerian," in *Herbs for the Mind: Depression, Stress, Memory Loss, and Insomnia* (New York: Guilford Press, 2000), 214–33.

Donath, F., et al., "Roots I: Critical Evaluation of the Effect of Valerian Extract on Sleep Structure and Sleep Quality," *Pharmacopsychiatry* 33 (2000): 47–53.

Dorn, M., "Valerian Versus Oxazepam: Efficacy and Tolerability in Nonorganic and Nonpsychiatric Insomniacs: A Randomized, Double-Blind, Clinical Comparative Study [in German]," *Forschende Komplementärmedizin und Klassische Naturheilkunde* 7 (2000): 79–84.

Russo, E. B., "Valerian," in *Handbook of Psychotropic Herbs: A Scientific Analysis of Herbal Remedies in Psychiatric Conditions* (Binghamton, N.Y.: Haworth Press, 2001), 95–106.

Vorbach, E. U., R. Gortelmeyer, and J. Bruning, "Treatment of Insomnia: Effectiveness and Tolerance of a Valerian Extract," *Psychopharmakotherapie* 3 (1996): 109–15.

CHAPTER 21

Amen, D. G., "Attention Deficit Disorder: A Guide for Primary Care Physicians," *Primary Psychiatry* 5, no. 7 (July 1998): 76–85.

———, *Change Your Brain, Change Your Life* (New York: Three Rivers Press, 1999).

———, *Images of Human Behavior, A Brain SPECT Atlas* (Newport Beach, Calif.: Mindworks Press, 2001).

———, *Healing ADD: The Breakthrough Program That Allows You to See and Heal the Six Types of Attention Deficit Disorder* (New York: G.P. Putnam and Sons, 2001).

Amen, D. G., with L. Routh, *Healing Anxiety and Depression* (New York: Putnam, 2003).

APPENDIX

Amen, D. G., "Why Don't Psychiatrists Look at the Brain: The Case for the Greater Use of SPECT Imaging in Neuropsychiatry," *Neuropsychiatry Reviews* 2, no. 1 (February 2001): 19–21.

Bonte, F. J., et al., "Brain Blood Flow in the Dementias: SPECT with Histopathologic Correlation in 54 Patients," *Radiology* 202 (1997): 793–97.

"Brain Perfusion Single Photon Emission Computed Tomography (SPECT) Using Tc-99m Radiopharmaceuticals 2.0. Approved 1999," in *Society of Nuclear Medicine Procedure Guidelines Manual* (June 2002).

Camargo, E. E., "Brain SPECT in Neurology and Psychiatry," *Journal of Nuclear Medicine* 42, no. 4 (April 2001): 611–23.

Chiron, C., et al., "Changes in Regional Cerebral Blood Flow During Brain Maturation in Children and Adolescents," *Journal of Nuclear Medicine* 33, no. 5 (May 1992): 696–703.

George, M. S., *Neuroactivation and Neuroimaging with SPECT* (New York: Springer-Verlag, 1991).

Report of the Therapeutics and Technology Assessment Subcommittee of the American Academy of Neurology: Assesment of Brain SPECT 46 (1996): 278–85.

Villanueva-Meyer, J., et al., "Cerebral Blood Flow During a Mental Activation Task: Responses in Normal Subjects and in Early Alzheimer Disease Patients," *Alasbimn Journal* 1, no. 3 (2000): http://www.alasbimnjournal.cl/revistas/3/villanuevaa.htm.

ACKNOWLEDGMENTS

I am grateful to many people who have been instrumental in the creation of this book, especially all of the patients and professionals who have come my way and taught me about the many different ways to optimize and heal the brain. The staff at Amen Clinics has been of help and tremendous support during this process, including David Bennett, Breanne Amen, Jesse Payne, Niccole Miller, Heather Manley, Chris Hanks, Mary Ann Wallner, Ronnette Leonard, and all the members of our research team, including Jill Prunella and Yalda Shafihie. A special thanks to my colleagues who provided input to the book, especially Sara Gilman, Earl Henslin, J. J. Virgin, John Trudeau, René Thomas, and Mark Kosins. I also wish to thank my wonderful, fun, and loving literary team at Harmony Books, Shaye Areheart, Kim Meisner, and Tara Gilbride. I am grateful to my literary agent Faith Hamlin, who is a constant source of strength, support, love, honesty, and encouragement.

INDEX

ABOUT THE AUTHOR

DANIEL G. AMEN, M.D., is a clinical neuroscientist, psychiatrist, brain-imaging expert, and medical director of Amen Clinics in Newport Beach and Fairfield, California; Tacoma, Washington; and Reston, Virginia. He is a nationally recognized expert in the field of brain and behavior, lecturing to thousands of mental health professionals, judges, and lay audiences each year. His clinics have the world's largest database of brain images relating to behavior.

Dr. Amen is assistant clinical professor of psychiatry and human behavior at the University of California, Irvine, School of Medicine. He did his psychiatric training at the Walter Reed Army Medical Center in Washington, D.C. He has won writing and research awards from the American Psychiatric Association, the U.S. Army, and the Baltimore-D.C. Institute for Psychoanalysis. He has been elected to the status of Distinguished Fellowship in the American Psychiatric Association.

Dr. Amen's writings have been published around the world. He is the author of numerous professional and popular articles, twenty books, and a number of audio and video programs. His books have been translated into thirteen languages and include *Change Your Brain, Change Your Life*, a *New York Times* bestseller; *Healing ADD; Healing the Hardware of the Soul; Healing Anxiety and Depression* (with Dr. Lisa Routh); *Preventing Alzheimer's Disease* (with Dr. Rod Shankle); and *Sex on the Brain*.

Dr. Amen, together with the United Paramount Network and Leeza Gibbons, produced a show called *The Truth About Drinking* on alcohol education for teenagers, which won the Emmy award in 1999 for the Best Educational Television Show. In addition, Dr. Amen has appeared on *The Today Show*, CNN, *The View, 48 Hours, The Jane Pauley Show, HBO America Undercover: Small Town Ecstasy,* MSNBC, PAX, *Discovery Channel News: Inside the Mind of a Killer, The 700 Club* (on drug abuse), Discovery Channel's *Next Step*, ABC, NBC, and CBS News, and more than four hundred radio interviews worldwide. His print credits include *Newsweek, Parade, Bonkers, Science & Vie–France, McCall's, Ladies' Home Journal, Parenting,* and the *Wall Street Journal*. Dr. Amen writes a monthly column for *Men's Health* magazine titled "Head Check."

AMEN CLINICS, INC.

Amen Clinics, Inc., was established in 1989 by Daniel G. Amen, M.D. The clinics specialize in innovative diagnosis and treatment planning for a wide variety of behavioral, learning, and emotional problems for children, teenagers, and adults. The clinics have an international reputation for evaluating brain-behavior problems, such as attention deficit disorder (ADD), depression, anxiety, school failure, brain trauma, obsessive-compulsive disorder, aggressiveness, cognitive decline, and brain toxicity from drugs or alcohol. Brain SPECT imaging is performed in the clinics. Amen Clinics has the world's largest database of brain scans for behavioral problems in the world.

The clinics welcome referrals from physicians, psychologists, social workers, marriage and family therapists, drug and alcohol counselors, and individual clients.

Amen Clinics, Inc., Newport Beach
4019 Westerly Place, Suite 100
Newport Beach, CA 92660
(949) 266-3700

Amen Clinics, Inc., Fairfield
350 Chadbourne Road
Fairfield, CA 94585
(707) 429-7181

Amen Clinics, Inc., Northwest
3315 South 23rd Street
Tacoma, WA 98405
(253) 779-HOPE

Amen Clinics, Inc., D.C.
1875 Campus Commons Drive
Reston, VA 20191
(703) 860-5600

www.amenclinic.com

AMENCLINIC.COM

Amenclinic.com is an educational interactive website geared toward mental health and medical professionals, educators, students, and the general public. It contains a wealth of information to help you learn about the clinics and the brain. The site contains more than three hundred color brain SPECT images, hundreds of scientific abstracts on brain SPECT imaging for psychiatry, a brain puzzle, and much, much more.

VIEW MORE THAN THREE HUNDRED ASTONISHING COLOR 3D BRAIN SPECT IMAGES ON:

Aggression
Attention deficit disorder, including the six subtypes
Dementia and cognitive decline
Drug abuse
PMS
Anxiety disorders
Brain trauma
Depression
Obsessive-compulsive disorder
Stroke
Seizures

ALSO BY DANIEL G. AMEN, M.D.

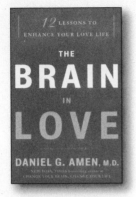

The Brain in Love
12 Lessons to Enhance Your Love Life
ISBN 978-0-307-58789-3
$14.00 paper (Canada: $17.99)

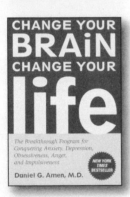

Change Your Brain, Change Your Life
The Breakthrough Program for Conquering
Anxiety, Depression, Obsessiveness, Anger, and
Impulsiveness
ISBN 978-0-8129-2998-0
$16.00 paper (Canada: $19.95)

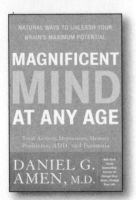

Magnificent Mind at Any Age
Natural Ways to Unleash Your Brain's Maximum
Potential
ISBN 978-0-307-33909-6
$24.95 hardcover (Canada: $27.95)

**COMING FROM
POTTER STYLE
IN SPRING 2010!**

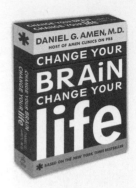

Change Your Brain, Change Your Life Deck
ISBN 978-0-307-46457-6
$14.99 deck (Canada: $18.99)

**COMING FROM
HARMONY BOOKS
IN SPRING 2010!**

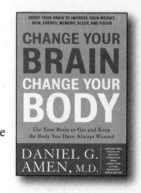

Change Your Brain, Change Your Body
Use Your Brain to Get and Keep the Body You Have
Always Wanted
ISBN 978-0-307-46357-9
$25.99 hardcover (Canada: $32.99)

Available wherever books are sold